VIROLOGY RESEARCH PROGRESS

# EBOLA

# ESSENTIALS, RESPONSE EFFORTS, AND PREVENTION ISSUES

# VIROLOGY RESEARCH PROGRESS

Additional books in this series can be found on Nova's website under the Series tab.

Additional e-books in this series can be found on Nova's website under the e-book tab.

VIROLOGY RESEARCH PROGRESS

# EBOLA

# ESSENTIALS, RESPONSE EFFORTS, AND PREVENTION ISSUES

MARYANN COLE
EDITOR

nova publishers
*New York*

**Library of Congress Cataloging-in-Publication Data**

ISBN: 978-1-63482-253-4

*Published by Nova Science Publishers, Inc. † New York*

# CONTENTS

# PREFACE

The Ebola virus is named after the Ebola River, near where the virus was discovered in 1976 in Zaire, now known as the Democratic Republic of the Congo (DRC). It is in the filovirus family, so called because of its filamentous shape. EVD is also known as Ebola hemorrhagic fever. The disease sometimes causes hemorrhage (i.e., bleeding) from body openings, but this symptom is not consistent. Five strains of Ebola virus have been identified. This book discusses the essentials, response efforts, and prevention issues involved with the Ebola virus.

Chapter 1 - In March 2014, global health officials recognized an outbreak of Ebola virus disease (EVD) in Guinea, West Africa. In retrospect, officials determined that the outbreak began in December 2013, and spread to the adjacent countries of Liberia and Sierra Leone. In September 2014, the U.S. Centers for Disease Control and Prevention (CDC) confirmed the first EVD case diagnosed in the United States, heightening concerns among some who fear the disease could spread in American communities. This report discusses EVD in general, including symptoms, modes of transmission, incubation period, and treatments. Unless otherwise cited, information in this report is drawn from Ebola information pages of CDC and the World Health Organization (WHO).

Chapter 2 - In March 2014, an Ebola Virus Disease (EVD) outbreak was reported in Guinea, West Africa. The outbreak is the first in West Africa and has caused an unprecedented number of cases and deaths. The outbreak is continuing to spread in Guinea, Sierra Leone, and Liberia (the "affected countries"); it has been contained in Nigeria and Senegal, and has been detected in Mali. As of October 22, 2014, more than 10,000 people have contracted EVD, more than half of whom have died.

Until October 2014, no secondary EVD cases had occurred outside of Africa. That month, health workers in Spain and the United States contracted EVD cases while providing care for Ebola patients. Other factors make this outbreak unique, including

- its introduction into West Africa;
- multi-country outbreaks occurring simultaneously;
- disease transmission within urban areas; and
- an unprecedented scale and pace of transmission.

In the aggregate, between 1976, when Ebola was first identified, through 2012, there were 2,387 cases, including 1,590 deaths, all in Central and East Africa. The number of Ebola cases in this outbreak is four times higher than the combined total of all prior outbreaks, and the number of cases is doubling monthly. The U.S. Centers for Disease Control and Prevention (CDC) and the World Health Organization (WHO) have projected an exponential increase in cases. WHO estimated that by the end of November, some 20,000 people may contract Ebola; CDC estimated that "without additional interventions or changes in community behavior," up to 1.4 million could contract EVD in Liberia and Sierra Leone by January 2015. CDC indicates, however, that the outbreak may not reach such proportions since responses are intensifying. In Liberia, for example, improvements in burial practices have resulted in roughly 85% of all bodies being collected within 24 hours of being reported to national officials.

In an August 2014 report, WHO estimated that it would cost roughly $500 million to contain the outbreak by January. In September, international responses accelerated. The United Nations (U.N.) established the United Nations Mission for Ebola Emergency Response (UNMEER) "to utilize the assets of all relevant U.N. agencies" to address the health and broader social impacts of the outbreak. A proposed U.N. response would cost roughly $1 billion, about half of which would be aimed at addressing health impacts.

The United States is the leading funder of the international Ebola response, and its financial support is growing. As of October 25, almost 900 U.S. government personnel had deployed to the region, and some 4,000 military personnel will be deployed to the region. The U.S. Agency for International Development (USAID) reports that as of October 22, U.S. funding for EVD responses totaled $344.6 million. In addition, the Department of Defense (DOD) is planning to spend more than $1 billion on EVD activities in West Africa. On October 17, President Obama established an Ebola Czar to coordinate U.S. domestic and global responses to the Ebola outbreak.

Some global health experts have criticized the U.S. and international response to the Ebola outbreak, decrying the pace and scale of assistance. The limited impact of U.S. and international responses to the Ebola outbreak has raised several questions regarding global health governance structures, international commitment to bolstering pandemic preparedness and response capacity in poor countries, and global support for strengthening health systems. The international community lacks a rapid response team of health professionals prepared to address health emergencies like the ongoing West African Ebola outbreak. Debates about whether WHO should have such capacity have been at the heart of recent WHO reform debates. While deliberating the appropriate response to ongoing Ebola outbreak, Congress is likely to discuss the breadth of health, social, economic, development, and security challenges that this outbreak is causing, as well as how U.S. global health aid is apportioned. This report focuses on the health impacts of the outbreak and discusses U.S. and international responses to those health challenges.

Chapter 3 - Throughout 2014, an outbreak of Ebola virus disease (EVD) has outpaced the efforts of health workers trying to contain it in three West African countries: Guinea, Liberia, and Sierra Leone. (These are often referred to as "affected countries" or "countries with widespread transmission." In mid-November, 2014, Ebola transmission also occurred for the second time in neighboring Mali. The extent of spread in Mali remains to be seen.) EVD cases have been imported to other countries, including the United States, where two nurses were infected while caring for a patient who had traveled from Liberia.

Members of Congress and the public have considered ways to prevent the entry and spread of EVD in the United States. Official recommendations have seemed to conflict at times. In part this reflects the evolution of officials' understanding of this new threat and the scientific and technical aspects of its control. In addition, under the nation's federalist governance structure, the federal and state governments are empowered to take measures to control communicable diseases, and have addressed some aspects of the Ebola threat in varied ways. In the United States and abroad, public concern about the spread of Ebola also may have shaped policymakers' decisions as well.

Chapter 4 - This is the Statement of Dr. Thomas R. Frieden, Director, Centers for Disease Control and Prevention.

Chapter 5 - This is the Testimony of Dr. Anthony S. Fauci, Director, National Institute of Allergy and Infectious Diseases.

Chapter 6 - This is the Statement of Sylvia Burwell, Secretary, U.S. Department of Health and Human Services.

Chapter 7 - This is the Statement of Jeh Johnson, Secretary, U.S. Department of Homeland Security.

Chapter 8 - Several West African countries are currently grappling with an unprecedented outbreak of Ebola virus disease (EVD). Here in the United States, where Ebola is not endemic, a handful of EVD cases have been diagnosed, and domestic transmission of the virus has occurred in only two cases to date. This report provides a brief overview of selected legal issues regarding measures to prevent transmission of Ebola virus and the civil rights of individuals affected by the disease.

Quarantine and isolation are restrictions on a person's movement, imposed to prevent the spread of contagious disease. The federal government has jurisdiction over interstate and border quarantine, carried out by the Centers for Disease Control and Prevention (CDC). However, primary quarantine authority typically resides with state health departments and health officials. Every state has the authority to pass and enforce quarantine laws as an exercise of its police powers, but these laws may vary widely by state. State and federal quarantine or isolation orders may be subject to suits alleging inadequate due process or violations of equal protection, but modern legal challenges to quarantine and isolation orders are not extensive.

In addition to the quarantine and isolation of persons within the United States, some have proposed limiting the entry of persons traveling to the United States from countries experiencing high rates of EVD transmission. Federal agencies' authority to restrict or regulate the entry into the United States of persons who are suspected of carrying Ebola virus or other communicable diseases depends largely upon whether the person is a foreign or U.S. national. Aliens who have been determined to carry Ebola virus may be denied entry, but the health-related grounds for exclusion do not apply to most lawful permanent residents who briefly travel abroad. U.S. citizens abroad may enjoy a constitutional right to reenter the country, in which case the government would be required, at a minimum, to overcome a heavier burden to justify a reentry restriction.

Proposals to restrict air travel to and from affected countries—regardless of citizenship—have also been discussed. The Federal Aviation Administration (FAA) has acknowledged its authority to restrict the use of U.S. airspace, but has cautioned that decisions made on a public health basis would involve other federal agencies. Additionally, the Do Not Board (DNB) list provides a mechanism for U.S. and international health officials to request that specific persons be restricted from boarding commercial aircraft to the United States, on the basis that those persons present a public health risk. Independently, airlines may reserve the right to deny transportation to passengers who may pose a safety risk, but must act consistent with federal nondiscrimination laws.

The use of these measures to contain the spread of Ebola may raise a classic civil rights issue: to what extent can an individual's liberty be curtailed to advance the common good? In addition to the constitutional issues noted above, discrimination against individuals with an infectious disease may be covered by Section 504 of the Rehabilitation Act, the Americans with Disabilities Act (ADA), or the Air Carrier Access Act (ACAA). While quarantine and isolation effectively minimize Ebola exposure, they may also raise various employment concerns, particularly for those workers who fear losing their jobs or wages if they are forced to comply with a quarantine or isolation order. Infected workers may also be protected under the Family and Medical Leave Act (FMLA) if it can be established that they have a serious health condition, and employers whose employees could face workplace exposure to Ebola virus may be obligated to comply with applicable Occupational Safety and Health Administration (OSHA) requirements.

Chapter 9 - In the wake of increasing fears about the spread of highly contagious diseases, federal, state, and local governments have become increasingly aware of the need for a comprehensive public health response to such events. An effective response could include the quarantine of persons exposed to infectious biological agents that are naturally occurring or released during a terrorist attack, the isolation of infected persons, and the quarantine of certain cities or neighborhoods.

The public health authority of the states derives from the police powers granted by their constitutions and reserved to them by the Tenth Amendment to the U.S. Constitution. The authority of the federal government to prescribe quarantine and other health measures is based on the Commerce Clause, which gives Congress exclusive authority to regulate interstate and foreign commerce. Thus, state and local governments have the primary authority to control the spread of dangerous diseases within their jurisdictions, and the federal government has authority to quarantine and impose other health measures to prevent the spread of diseases from foreign countries and between states. In addition, the federal government may assist state efforts to prevent the spread of communicable diseases if requested by a state or if state efforts are inadequate to halt the spread of disease.

This report provides an overview of federal and state public health laws as they relate to the quarantine and isolation of individuals and a discussion of constitutional issues that may be raised should individual liberties be restricted in a quarantine or isolation situation.

In: Ebola
Editor: MaryAnn Cole
ISBN: 978-1-63482-253-4


*Chapter 1*

# EBOLA: BASICS ABOUT THE DISEASE*

*Sarah A. Lister*

In March 2014, global health officials recognized an outbreak of Ebola virus disease (EVD) in Guinea, West Africa. In retrospect, officials determined that the outbreak began in December 2013, and spread to the adjacent countries of Liberia and Sierra Leone. In September 2014, the U.S. Centers for Disease Control and Prevention (CDC) confirmed the first EVD case diagnosed in the United States,[1] heightening concerns among some who fear the disease could spread in American communities.[2] This report discusses EVD in general, including symptoms, modes of transmission, incubation period, and treatments. Unless otherwise cited, information in this report is drawn from Ebola information pages of CDC[3] and the World Health Organization (WHO).[4]

## THE EBOLA VIRUS AND EVD

The Ebola virus is named after the Ebola River, near where the virus was discovered in 1976 in Zaire, now known as the Democratic Republic of the Congo (DRC). It is in the filovirus family, so called because of its filamentous

* This is an edited, reformatted and augmented version of a Congressional Research Service publication R43750, prepared for Members and Committees of Congress, dated October 3, 2014.

shape. EVD is also known as Ebola hemorrhagic fever. The disease sometimes causes hemorrhage (i.e., bleeding) from body openings, but this symptom is not consistent. Five strains of Ebola virus have been identified. The Zaire strain is responsible for the current outbreak in West Africa. A slightly different Zaire strain is responsible for a smaller unrelated outbreak now in the DRC.

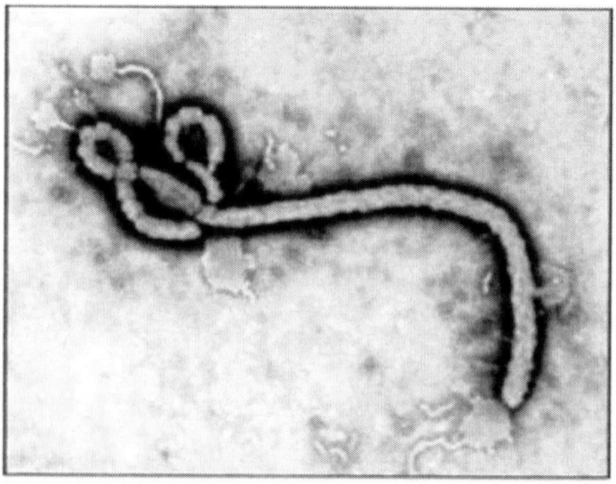

Source: Colorized transmission electron micrograph from CDC, Public Health Image Library, image #10815, http://phil.cdc.gov.

Figure 1. Ebola Virus Particle.

## TRANSMISSION

Ebola virus is thought to live in nonhuman animals in parts of Africa. Fruit bats are thought to be the most likely or most common animal reservoir for the virus. Humans may be exposed through contact with infected animals.

During an outbreak, EVD spreads through human-to-human transmission. Transmission requires direct contact with body fluids from an infected person or contaminated objects such as medical equipment. It cannot be spread through the air. Hence, EVD is not as easily transmitted as influenza or common cold viruses, which can be spread through the air. However, healthcare workers, family members, and others who care for EVD patients have a high risk of infection because they are in regular contact with infected body fluids.

In humans EVD has an incubation period—the time between exposure and onset of symptoms— from 2 to 21 days, with an average of 8 to10 days.

Individuals are not contagious, meaning they cannot transmit EVD to others, until symptoms are present. Those surviving infection may still have Ebola virus in their bodies and remain contagious for several months after infection, even when symptoms are no longer present. They can be tested for the presence of virus in order to maintain their quarantine until they are no longer contagious.

## SYMPTOMS AND DIAGNOSIS

The early symptoms of EVD are shared by many more common illnesses, complicating diagnosis.[5] Symptoms may include a high fever (greater than 38.6°C, or 101.5°F), severe headache, muscle pain, weakness, diarrhea, vomiting, abdominal (stomach) pain, and unexplained hemorrhage (bleeding or bruising).

Several laboratory tests are available to test patients for EVD. These tests may yield negative results within the first few days after symptoms appear. As a result, patients who have potentially been exposed to EVD and who show some of the symptoms above should be isolated, even if test results are negative, and retested a few days later.

**Isolation or Quarantine?**

Isolation is used to separate ill persons who have a contagious disease from others. It is often carried out in a healthcare setting.

Quarantine is used to separate and restrict the movement of well persons who may have been exposed to a contagious disease to see if they become ill. It is often carried out at home.

## DEATH RATES

EVD is known and widely feared for being exceptionally deadly. The case fatality rate (CFR), the percentage of infected individuals who do not survive, generally exceeds 50%, an extraordinarily high rate among infectious diseases. The true CFR is an inherent property of the infectious agent (in this case, the Ebola Zaire virus). However, the measured CFR is affected by the availability of vaccines and specific treatments, as well as general medical care, among other factors. Perhaps the most significant factor is how cases are counted; whether counts are limited, for example, to cases in which EVD is confirmed with a laboratory test, or to hospitalized patients, or to patients for whom an outcome (lived or died) is confirmed. Different approaches to case counting can affect the measured CFR considerably.

WHO analyzed CFRs for the current outbreak in West Africa, limiting its analysis to patients with confirmed outcomes. It found rates of about 70% in each of the severely affected countries— Guinea (70.7%), Liberia (72.3%), and Sierra Leone (69.0%). In all three countries, hospitalized patients in this group had somewhat lower CFRs (ranging from 61% to 67%) than patients who were not hospitalized.[6] Regardless of variations in measured rates, EVD is clearly a deadly disease.

## PREVENTING TRANSMISSION

Prevention of human-to-human transmission of Ebola virus requires avoiding contact with body fluids of those who are sick. As a result, EVD is not likely to be easily transmitted in community settings in the United States. However, caregivers, including family members and healthcare workers, face considerable risk of transmission. Barrier protections (called personal protective equipment or PPE), liberal disinfection of premises and facilities housing EVD patients, and careful handling of human remains and contaminated objects are essential.[7] In resource-constrained environments (such as in developing countries), consistent adherence to these practices can be hampered by shortages of personnel and supplies, and other factors. However, according to CDC, "virtually any hospital in the [United States] can do isolation for Ebola."[8]

## THERAPIES AND VACCINES

No specific therapy or vaccine against EVD is approved by the U.S. Food and Drug Administration (FDA) for use in the United States, or is available elsewhere in the world. However, for more than a decade the U.S. government has funded research and development of specific therapies (such as antiviral drugs) and vaccines against EVD for military force protection and domestic biodefense purposes. Given the current outbreak, pharmaceutical companies,

FDA, and other federal agencies have accelerated their work on some promising products.[9] Some products are or may soon be available for investigational use (i.e., in clinical trials) both domestically and abroad.

WHO assumes that EVD-specific therapies and vaccines will not be available in sufficient time or amount to quell the current outbreak. It urges continued aggressive efforts to stop ongoing transmission through contact tracing (i.e., identifying and monitoring all individuals who may have been exposed to an infected patient) and use of protective measures.[10]

Non-EVD-specific treatments include fluids (orally or intravenously) to maintain hydration, and blood transfusions to counter blood loss from hemorrhagic symptoms. Transfusions of blood, serum, or plasma from EVD survivors have been given to some victims in order to provide antibodies from the survivors. The effectiveness of this approach has not been demonstrated.[11]

Testing unproven therapies in the midst of an outbreak raises technical and ethical concerns. A WHO committee has said that the use of investigational products is warranted for the current outbreak.[12] Experts disagree about the particulars of such use, however. For example, some say that in order to understand whether an investigational product is effective, it must be studied by comparing outcomes of groups of people who receive the product, and groups who receive a non-therapeutic drug or vaccine (i.e., a placebo) instead. Others feel that placebo comparisons are not necessary, arguing that if a given investigational product were effective, it would be evident in how it lowered the normally high case fatality rate of EVD, and more people would be able to benefit from it.[13] This issue often arises when clinical trials are carried out in developing countries; the path(s) chosen in deploying investigational products for EVD in West Africa will be examined in order to inform the response to outbreaks of EVD and other diseases in the future.

## OUTBREAK MODELS AND PROJECTIONS

Guinea, Liberia, and Sierra Leone, countries without prior experience with EVD, have been severely affected by the current outbreak. In late summer case counts in the three countries rose precipitously. On September 22, WHO warned that "[u]nless Ebola control measures in west Africa are enhanced quickly, ... numbers will continue to climb exponentially, and more than [20,000] people will have been infected by early November.... "[14]

The same week, CDC authors published outbreak projections for Liberia and Sierra Leone. The model found that without further interventions to slow the outbreak (a worst case scenario), the case count in the two countries could reach 1.4 million by January 20, 2015. Conversely, if 70% of EVD patients were effectively isolated going forward, the outbreak in both countries would be almost controlled by that same date.[15]

In light of concerns raised by the introduction of EVD into the United States, the CDC Director has said that these concerns can best be alleviated by controlling the outbreak in West Africa.[16]

## End Notes

[1] Centers for Disease Control and Prevention (CDC), "CDC and Texas Health Department Confirm First Ebola Case Diagnosed in the U.S.," press release, September 30, 2014,

[2] CRS Report IN10126, Safe at Home? Letting Ebola-Stricken Americans Return, by Sarah A. Lister.

[3] Centers for Disease Control and Prevention (CDC), "Ebola virus disease," http://www.cdc.gov/vhf/ebola/index.html.

[4] World Health Organization (WHO), "Ebola virus disease," http://www.who. int/csr/ disease/ ebola/en/.

[5] See for example Lauran Neergard and Paul J. Weber, "U.S. Hospital Sent Ebola-infected Patient Home," Associated Press, October 2, 2014, discussing initial failure of providers in a Dallas hospital to diagnose EVD in a patient.

[6] WHO Ebola Response Team, "Ebola Virus Disease in West Africa—The First 9 Months of the Epidemic and Forward Projections," NEJM, September 23, 2014, Table 2, p. 11, http://www.nejm.org.

[7] See for example CDC, "Ebola Virus Disease: Prevention," http://www.cdc.gov/vhf/ebola/ prevention/index.html.

[8] Comments of CDC Director Tom Frieden, "CDC Confirms First Ebola Case Diagnosed in the United States," Press Briefing Transcript, September 30, 2014, http://www.cdc.gov/ media/ archives.htm.

[9] FDA, "2014 Ebola Outbreak in West Africa," http://www.fda.gov/Emergency Prepared ness/Counterterrorism/ MedicalCountermeasures/ucm410308.htm; and CRS, Availability of Treatments for the Ebola Virus Outbreak in West Africa, memorandum for general distribution, September 12, 2014, by Frank Gottron, 7-5854, Sarah A. Lister, 7-7320, and Susan Thaul, 7-0562. Contact authors for a copy.

[10] WHO, Ebola Response Roadmap, August 28, 2014, Geneva, Switzerland, http://www.who. int/csr/disease/ebola/ ebola-response-roadmap/en/.

[11] WHO, "Experimental Therapies: Growing Interest in the Use of Whole Blood or Plasma from Recovered Ebola Patients (Convalescent Therapies)," September 26, 2014, http://who.int/mediacentre/news/ebola/26-september-2014/ en/.

[12] WHO, "Ethical Considerations for Use of Unregistered Interventions for Ebola Virus Disease: Report of an Advisory Panel to WHO," August 17, 2014, http://www.who.int/csr/resources/ publications/ebola/ethical-considerations/en/.

[13] See for example Kai Kupferschmidt, "Ebola Vaccine Tests Needlessly Delayed, Researchers Claim," Science magazine, September 29, 2014, http://news.sciencemag.org/category/ africa.

[14] WHO, "Study Warns Swift Action Needed to Curb Exponential Climb in Ebola Outbreak," press release, September 22, 2014, referring to the NEJM article at footnote 6, http://who.int/mediacentre/news/releases/2014/ebola-study/en/.

[15] Martin I. Meltzer et al., “Estimating the Future Number of Cases in the Ebola Epidemic—Liberia and Sierra Leone, 2014–2015,” MMWR, vol. 63, Supplement, no. 3 (September 26, 2014), pp. 1-14, http://www.cdc.gov/mmwr/.

[16] See for example comments of CDC Director Tom Frieden, “ CDC Confirms First Ebola Case Diagnosed in the United States,” Press Briefing Transcript, September 30, 2014, http://www.cdc.gov/media/archives.htm.

In: Ebola
Editor: MaryAnn Cole

ISBN: 978-1-63482-253-4


*Chapter 2*

# U.S. AND INTERNATIONAL HEALTH RESPONSES TO THE EBOLA OUTBREAK IN WEST AFRICA*

***Tiaji Salaam-Blyther***

## SUMMARY

In March 2014, an Ebola Virus Disease (EVD) outbreak was reported in Guinea, West Africa. The outbreak is the first in West Africa and has caused an unprecedented number of cases and deaths. The outbreak is continuing to spread in Guinea, Sierra Leone, and Liberia (the "affected countries"); it has been contained in Nigeria and Senegal, and has been detected in Mali. As of October 22, 2014, more than 10,000 people have contracted EVD, more than half of whom have died.

Until October 2014, no secondary EVD cases had occurred outside of Africa. That month, health workers in Spain and the United States contracted EVD cases while providing care for Ebola patients. Other factors make this outbreak unique, including

- its introduction into West Africa;
- multi-country outbreaks occurring simultaneously;
- disease transmission within urban areas; and
- an unprecedented scale and pace of transmission.

* This is an edited, reformatted and augmented version of a Congressional Research Service publication, No. R43697, dated October 29, 2014.

In the aggregate, between 1976, when Ebola was first identified, through 2012, there were 2,387 cases, including 1,590 deaths, all in Central and East Africa. The number of Ebola cases in this outbreak is four times higher than the combined total of all prior outbreaks, and the number of cases is doubling monthly. The U.S. Centers for Disease Control and Prevention (CDC) and the World Health Organization (WHO) have projected an exponential increase in cases. WHO estimated that by the end of November, some 20,000 people may contract Ebola; CDC estimated that "without additional interventions or changes in community behavior," up to 1.4 million could contract EVD in Liberia and Sierra Leone by January 2015. CDC indicates, however, that the outbreak may not reach such proportions since responses are intensifying. In Liberia, for example, improvements in burial practices have resulted in roughly 85% of all bodies being collected within 24 hours of being reported to national officials.

In an August 2014 report, WHO estimated that it would cost roughly $500 million to contain the outbreak by January. In September, international responses accelerated. The United Nations (U.N.) established the United Nations Mission for Ebola Emergency Response (UNMEER) "to utilize the assets of all relevant U.N. agencies" to address the health and broader social impacts of the outbreak. A proposed U.N. response would cost roughly $1 billion, about half of which would be aimed at addressing health impacts.

The United States is the leading funder of the international Ebola response, and its financial support is growing. As of October 25, almost 900 U.S. government personnel had deployed to the region, and some 4,000 military personnel will be deployed to the region. The U.S. Agency for International Development (USAID) reports that as of October 22, U.S. funding for EVD responses totaled $344.6 million. In addition, the Department of Defense (DOD) is planning to spend more than $1 billion on EVD activities in West Africa. On October 17, President Obama established an Ebola Czar to coordinate U.S. domestic and global responses to the Ebola outbreak.

Some global health experts have criticized the U.S. and international response to the Ebola outbreak, decrying the pace and scale of assistance. The limited impact of U.S. and international responses to the Ebola outbreak has raised several questions regarding global health governance structures, international commitment to bolstering pandemic preparedness and response capacity in poor countries, and global support for strengthening health systems. The international community lacks a rapid response team of health professionals prepared to address health emergencies like the ongoing West African Ebola outbreak. Debates about whether WHO should have such capacity have been at the heart of recent WHO reform debates. While deliberating the appropriate response to ongoing Ebola outbreak, Congress is likely to discuss the breadth of health, social, economic, development, and security challenges that this outbreak is causing, as well as how U.S. global health aid is apportioned. This report focuses on the health impacts of the outbreak and discusses U.S. and international responses to those health challenges.

## BACKGROUND

Ebola virus disease (Ebola, or EVD) is a severe, often fatal disease that was first detected in the Democratic Republic of the Congo (DRC) in 1976.[1] Originating in animals, EVD is spread to and among humans through contact with the blood, other bodily fluids, organs, and corpses of those infected. It is not transmitted through the air, and the World Health Organization (WHO) maintains that there is minimal risk of contracting EVD on a plane,[2] though most airlines have suspended flights to and from the affected countries.[3]

In March 2014, an EVD outbreak was reported in Guinea, West Africa. The outbreak is the first in West Africa and has become the largest, most persistent ever documented. The outbreak is continuing to spread in Guinea, Sierra Leone, and Liberia ("affected countries") and has ended in Nigeria and Senegal, after having infected 20 people in Nigeria and one in Senegal. As of late October, nearly 10,000 people have contracted EVD, of whom almost 5,000 have died (**Figure 1**). WHO regularly updates EVD cases at http://www.who.int/ebola.

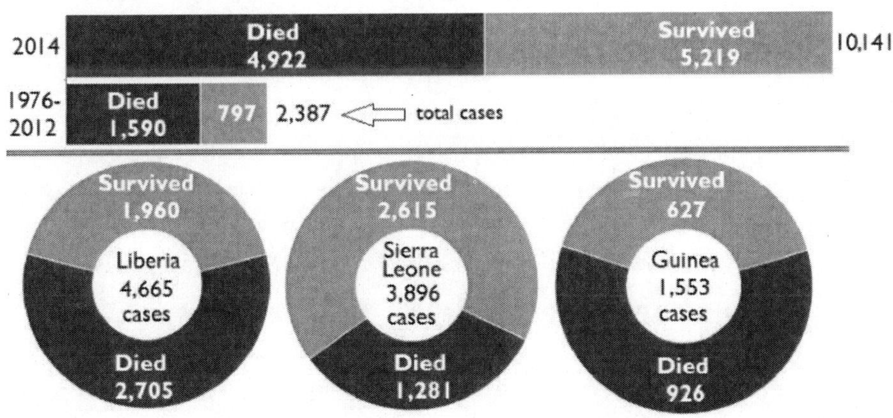


Source: Created by CRS Global Health Specialist Tiaji Salaam-Blyther from WHO data.

Figure 1. Ebola Outbreaks: 1976-2014, as Reported on October 22, 2014.

Due to inadequate disease surveillance capacities in the region, WHO estimates that actual cases may be two to four times higher than reported.[4] Some health experts are concerned that the weak surveillance systems in neighboring countries may miss EVD cases. On October 23, Mali reported its first EVD case and some suspect that Cote d'Ivoire may have undetected cases.[5] WHO is reportedly sending a team to Mali to help with clinical management, epidemiology, contact tracing and social mobilization.

## Ebola Care and Treatment

There are no drugs proven to prevent or treat EVD, though efforts are underway to develop them. In October, press reports indicated that WHO planned to begin testing two Ebola vaccines in January on some 20,000 health workers and other volunteers. The organization also indicated that a treatment might be available for use in Liberia by early November.[6] In the absence of specific treatments, health practitioners treat EVD symptoms with supportive care, which can reduce the fatality rate. Spread of the disease can be limited through the use of disease surveillance and containment measures. WHO has released manuals that outline appropriate patient care, management of contaminated objects, safe burial practices, and diagnostic protocol.[7] These measures successfully contained all the previous Ebola outbreaks.

## Distinguishing Factors

The Ebola virus that is circulating in West Africa is not new. Health experts are familiar with methods to treat and contain it. The disease is spreading quickly, however, because the health systems in the affected countries are ill-equipped to implement requisite disease containment and surveillance measures. Key factors that distinguish this outbreak from previous EVD outbreaks include the following:

### *Emergence in West Africa*

Prior to the current outbreak in Guinea, Liberia, and Sierra Leone (affected countries), EVD outbreaks were concentrated in the DRC, Gabon, Sudan South Sudan, and Uganda (**Figure 3**).

### *Simultaneous Multi-Country Outbreaks*

Disease transmission along the shared borders of Guinea, Liberia, and Sierra Leone has been intense and despite efforts to detect the disease at the borders, people infected with Ebola have imported the disease into other countries. Contact tracing and disease containment have halted the spread in Senegal and Nigeria where the outbreak ended on October 17 and 19, respectively. In Nigeria, an imported case resulted in an outbreak that infected 20 people and killed eight. A single imported case in Senegal was contained to the index case. WHO is investigating a new EVD case in Mali.

Until October, no EVD cases outside of Africa resulted in secondary cases. In that month, health workers in the United States and Spain contracted EVD while caring for EVD patients. No additional cases have been reported from the health workers. No other reports have emerged of EVD spreading in other countries where EVD patients have been evacuated.

### *Cases in Urban Areas*

Previous outbreaks were confined to rural and forested areas, whereas the current outbreak is spreading in rural and urban settings alike. Responders are struggling to isolate cases and contain the outbreak in densely populated urban areas that lack sufficient access to clean water and sanitation and face severe shortages of health workers and clinics.

### *Scale and Pace of Transmission*

Ebola is spreading at an unprecedented rate in the affected countries. In Liberia, reported cases are doubling every 15-20 days and in Sierra Leone, reported cases are doubling every 30-40 days.[8] Health experts link the unabated spread of EVD in the affected countries to weak health systems.

## Unrelated, Ongoing Ebola Outbreak

A separate Ebola outbreak that is unrelated to the ongoing West Africa outbreak was detected in the DRC on August 24, 2014.[9] It reportedly began in late July or early August, when a woman contracted an EVD-like hemorrhagic fever after butchering a wild animal. She later died and infected several others. As of October 20, there have been 66 cases and 49 deaths in the DRC, including eight deaths among health workers. All but five of the 1,121 contacts have completed the 21-day follow-up period.[10] This is the seventh outbreak of EVD in the DRC since 1976.

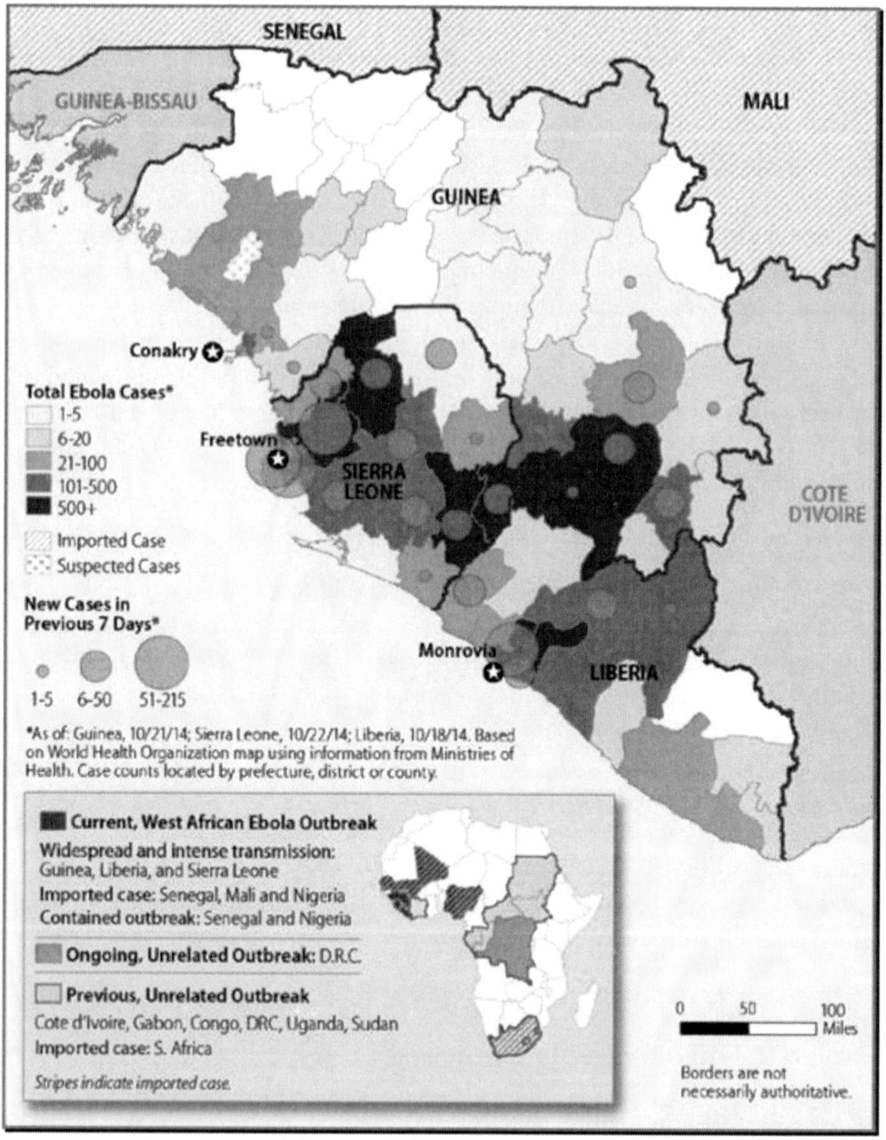


Source: Created by CRS Visual Information Specialist Amber Wilheim from WHO data.

Figure 2. Map of Current and Past Ebola Outbreaks.

## Congressional Actions

Congressional actions to address the outbreak have been accelerating. Several committees have convened hearings on the Ebola outbreak and in July and September 2014, U.S. Representative Karen Bass and Senator Christopher Coons introduced legislation recognizing the severe impacts and threats of the outbreak.[11]

Also in September, Congress enacted legislation (P.L. 113-164, Continuing Appropriations Resolution, 2015) that provided $88 million for the Ebola response: $30 million for CDC Ebola response activities in West Africa and $58 million for research and development of specific treatments and vaccines for Ebola.

Congress has also permitted the Department of Defense (DOD) to reprogram roughly $750 million of FY2014 Overseas Humanitarian Disaster and Civic Aid (OHDACA) funds to build 17 Ebola treatment units (ETUs) in Liberia and to support ongoing U.S. efforts in the region (see "Department of Defense").

# HEALTH SYSTEM CONSTRAINTS IN AFFECTED COUNTRIES

The health systems in the affected countries were already weak before the Ebola outbreak, and have become overwhelmed by the crisis. According to WHO, there are six components of a health system: (1) human resources; (2) governance and leadership; (3) financing; (4) commodities and supply chain networkers; (5) service delivery; and (6) information.[12] The affected countries face severe deficiencies in each of these areas and the outbreak is exacerbating these challenges.

This section describes how constraints in each component of the affected countries' health systems enable the virus to continue to spread. **Table 1** summarizes these issues.

**Table 1. Impact of Health System Deficiencies on Ebola Outbreak Containment**

| Governance | | Financing | Human Resources | Commodities | Service Delivery | Information |
|---|---|---|---|---|---|---|
| Description | Policies, strategies, and plans that inform the course of action a country will take to meet the health needs of its people. | Mechanisms used to fund health efforts and allocate resources. | The people who provide healthcare and support health delivery. | Goods that are used to provide healthcare. | The management and delivery of healthcare. | The collection, analysis, and dissemination of health statistics for planning and allocating health resources. |
| Impact of Health System Component Deficiency in Ebola Context | Slow initial government response to the Ebola outbreak and incapacity to implement national Ebola plans has diminished public confidence in political authorities and limited efforts to dispel rumors and fears about Ebola. | Insufficient financial resources to fund local responses and pay health personnel contribute to human resource and commodity shortages. | Shortages of not only health personnel, but also support staff like grave diggers and statisticians limit the ability to detect, prevent, and treat EVD cases. | Insufficient supply of protective equipment threatens the safety of healthcare workers (including community volunteers) and is associated with hospital- and clinic-based infections. | Many health facilities in Liberia and Sierra Leone remain closed due to staff shortages and other factors. | Limited capacity to conduct contact tracing and diagnosis calls into question the actual EVD cases and impedes efforts to detect, treat, and control the virus. |

Source: Created by CRS Global Health Specialist Tiaji Salaam-Blyther from WHO webpage on health systems, http://www.who.int/topics/ health_systems, and research on the Ebola outbreak.

## Governance and Leadership

The unabated spread of the outbreak in the affected countries has contributed to perceptions of government ineptitude. Mistrust of public officials has prompted many civilians to ignore or resist government responses. Reports of attacks on health workers and health facilities (run by nongovernmental organization and national health ministries alike) persist. The affected governments have used armed forces to enforce disease control measures and to quarantine neighborhoods, further deepening public resentment. Some have questioned the effectiveness of quarantines and criticized the measures, citing concerns about human rights, food scarcity, and possible unrest. Following criticisms by health experts and protests, Liberia and Sierra Leone have stopped quarantining some neighborhoods, though some quarantine zones remain. Despite concerns about quarantine practices, Sierra Leonean officials had characterized a three-day "Stay Home House to House" sensitization campaign a success, noting during which 92 bodies had been recovered and 56 Ebola cases were detected.[13]

## Financing

Per capita health spending in Guinea, Liberia, and Sierra Leone has been relatively low (Table 2), contributing to poor conditions of publicly-funded health facilities. Health workers and other government personnel often experience delays in compensation and benefits, contributing to absenteeism and human worker shortages. As the Ebola outbreak intensified, some health workers abandoned their posts, citing not only safety concerns (from lack of protective equipment) but also frustration over not receiving salaries. Several local staff at Ebola treatment units in Liberia had reportedly not been paid for three months.[14] Donors, including the United States, have since begun to offer financial aid to Liberia to support payment of health workers salaries and other financial incentives.

All of the outbreak-affected countries lack sufficient financial resources to fund their national Ebola response plans and need financial support. Several donors have pledged to provide support to the affected countries, though gaps persist (see "International Health Responses"). To meet the health and secondary effects of the outbreak, the United Nations estimates that it will cost Guinea $194 million, Liberia, $473 million, and Sierra Leone $220 million. Roughly half of these resources will be needed for addressing health needs.[15]

**Table 2. Selected Health System Financing Statistics, 2011**

| | % of Population Living on < $1 Daily | Health Personnel per 10,000 Pop. | Per Capita Gov. Health Spending | Gov. Health Budget as % of Total Gov. Spending |
|---|---|---|---|---|
| Guinea | 43.3% | not available | $15 | 6.8% |
| Liberia | 83.8% | 2.8 | $27 | 19.1% |
| Sierra Leone | 51.7% | 1.9 | $31 | 12.3% |
| Nigeria | 68.0% | 20.2 | $49 | 6.7% |
| Africa | 51.5% | 14.6 | $76 | 9.7% |
| World | 21.5% | 43.3 | $619 | 15.2% |

Source: Created by CRS Global Health Specialist Tiaji Salaam-Blyther from WHO, *World Health Statistics Report*, 2014.

Notes: Health personnel refers to doctors, nurses, and midwives.

## Human Resources

Due to severe shortages of health workers and clinics, the majority of people infected with Ebola in Liberia are without access to medical care and treatment. Inadequate access to health personnel and facilities is also a problem in Sierra Leone and Guinea. Human resource constraints and concerns about conditions in health centers are prompting people to care for the ill on their own, facilitating the spread of the virus. The shortage of medics and health facilities also means that people needing care for non-EVD related issues have nowhere to go.

Observers are troubled not only by inadequate access to Ebola care but also to the impact that clinic closures are having on broader health issues, particularly maternal and child health. Before the outbreak, maternal and child mortality rates in the EVD-affected countries were among the highest in the world (**Figure 3**). In 2012, roughly 26% of all maternal deaths in sub-Saharan Africa occurred in the four countries, where more than 46,000 women died from pregnancy-related complications (an average of 126 daily deaths).[16] Also in 2012, nearly one million children died in the affected countries before reaching their fifth birthday, accounting for roughly 30% of all under-five deaths in sub-Saharan Africa.[17] Most of these deaths could have been prevented with adequate access to vaccines, clean water and sanitation, and nutrition.

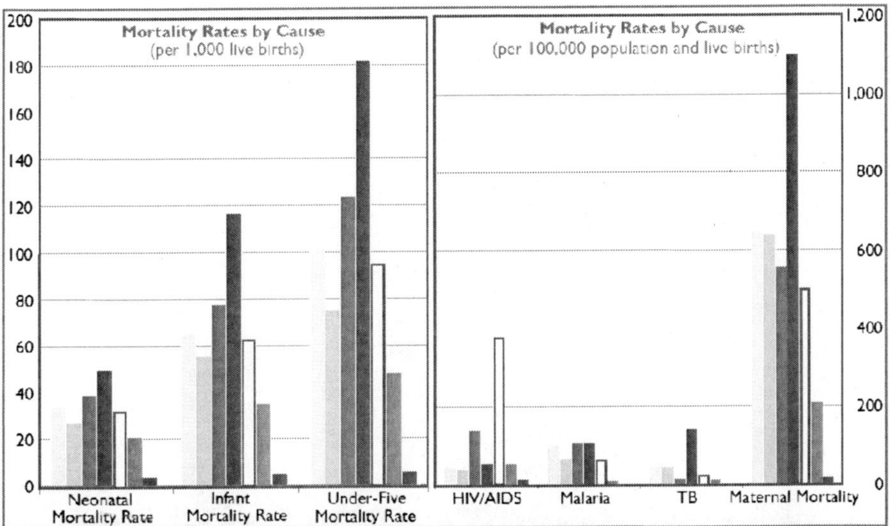


| Legend | HIV/AIDS | Malaria | TB | Maternal Mortality | Neonatal Morality | Infant Mortality | Under-Five Mortality Rate |
|---|---|---|---|---|---|---|---|
| | (per 100,000 population) | | | (per 100,000 live births) | (per 1,000 live births) | | |
| Guinea | 44 | 103 | 44 | 650 | 34 | 65 | 101 |
| Liberia | 40 | 69 | 46 | 640 | 27 | 56 | 75 |
| Nigeria | 142 | 108 | 16 | 560 | 39 | 78 | 124 |
| Sierra Leone | 55 | 108 | 143 | 1,100 | 50 | 117 | 182 |
| Africa | 377 | 63 | 26 | 500 | 32 | 63 | 95 |
| World | 56 | 11 | 13 | 210 | 21 | 35 | 48 |
| High Income Countries | 15 | 0 | 2 | 17 | 4 | 5 | 6 |

Source: Created by CRS Global Health Specialist Tiaji Salaam-Blyther from WHO, *World Health Statistics Report*, 2014.

Acronym: Tuberculosis (TB).

Notes: *Maternal mortality* refers to the death of a woman while pregnant or within 42 days of a terminated pregnancy from any cause related to or aggravated by the pregnancy or its mismanagement, but not from accidental or incidental causes. *Neonatal mortality* refers to the probability of dying during the first 28 days of life. *Infant Mortality* refers to the probability of dying within the first year of life. *Under-Five Mortality* refers to the probability of dying between before five years of age. All statistics collected in 2012, except maternal mortality rate, collected in 2013. In 2012 and 2013, the World Bank classified high-income countries as those with gross national incomes of $12,746 or more.

Figure 3. Health Statistics: Affected Countries, Africa, High-Income Countries, World.

Press reports indicate that some pregnant women are avoiding health facilities out of fear of contracting EVD in health settings. At the same time, many needing assistance during labor and delivery are unable to receive medical attention due to clinic closures and human resource constraints. According to the United Nations, "[m]ore people are now dying in Liberia from treatable ailments and common medical conditions than from Ebola."[18]

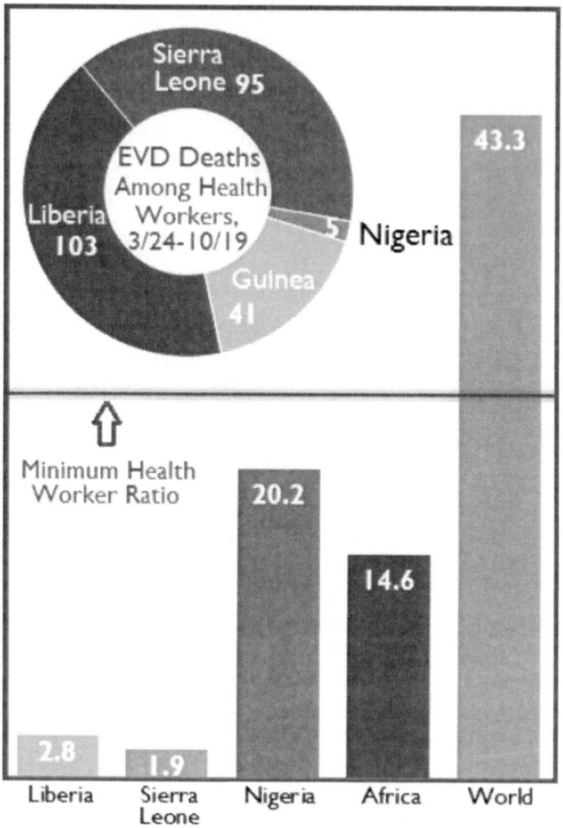


Source: Created by CRS Global Health Specialist Tiaji Salaam-Blyther from WHO, *World Health Statistics Report*, 2014 and WHO, *WHO: Ebola Response Roadmap Situation Report*, October 22, 2014.

Notes: Health personnel ratio data collected between 2006 and 2013.

Figure 4. Health Personnel Ratios and EVD Deaths Among Health Workers, (health personnel per 10,000 population, 2006-2013).

High maternal and child mortality rates in the affected countries are linked to the dearth of health workers in the affected countries. Between 2006 and 2013, Sierra Leone had only two doctors per 100,000 people, according to the WHO (**Figure 4**).[19] At an August 2014 congressional hearing, one witness testified that prior to the Ebola outbreak, Liberia had fewer than 200 doctors.[20]

After the outbreak, he estimated that about 50 doctors remained to provide clinical care, due in part to the evacuation of several expatriate doctors. EVD deaths among health workers have further diminished these staffing levels. On October 22, WHO reported that 443 health workers had contracted EVD, of whom 244 died.[21] More than 40% of these deaths occurred in Liberia. Sierra Leone and Liberia face shortages that are much more severe than Nigeria and the rest of the world.

Ebola control is labor- and resource-intensive, due to requisite surveillance and containment measures. WHO estimates, for example, that a facility treating 70 Ebola patients needs at least 250 healthcare workers.[22] In order to stop the spread of EVD, WHO estimated at the end of August 2014 that the affected countries would need more than 13,000 health workers to provide health care, contact tracing, and safe burial.[23] The plan estimated that roughly 5% of the health personnel would come from foreign countries and the rest would be comprised of national health staff. The affected countries do not have enough health personnel and countries are beginning to deploy medics to the region.

## Service Delivery

The Ebola outbreak has further diminished healthcare options in the affected countries. Many health facilities in Liberia and Sierra Leone are closed. Even before the outbreak, access to clinics was limited. The vast majority of health facilities are concentrated in urban areas and Ebola treatment centers are concentrated in high prevalence areas, leaving large swaths of the population without access to both general healthcare and Ebola-specific treatment. Due to limited access to clinics, the ill frequently travel great distances in search of healthcare, prompting most to wait until health complications are severe. Delayed health-seeking practices are reducing survival prospects among those sickened by Ebola and encumbering efforts to detect and contain the virus.

A variety of health services are needed to control the outbreak, including Ebola treatment centers, laboratories, contact tracing, and safe burial services. All of the affected countries face severe deficiencies in these areas. Most of the health services are unable to meet the demands and new ones are filled up as soon as they are opened. Patients turned away from treatment facilities typically return to their communities, often on public transportation, likely infecting several more people along the way. CDC estimates that fatality rates could be halved if people were able to access treatment and healthcare.[24]

Liberia faces the most severe treatment shortage. As of October 22, WHO estimated that it had only 23% of the beds it needed to treat those sickened by EVD (**Figure 5**). Treatment capacity is expected to improve with U.S. plans to support the construction of 27 ETUs in the country, 12 of which will be built by the Department of Defense (DOD).[25] Health experts are investigating a recent reduction in people seeking Ebola care in Liberia, reportedly leaving some beds vacant.[26]

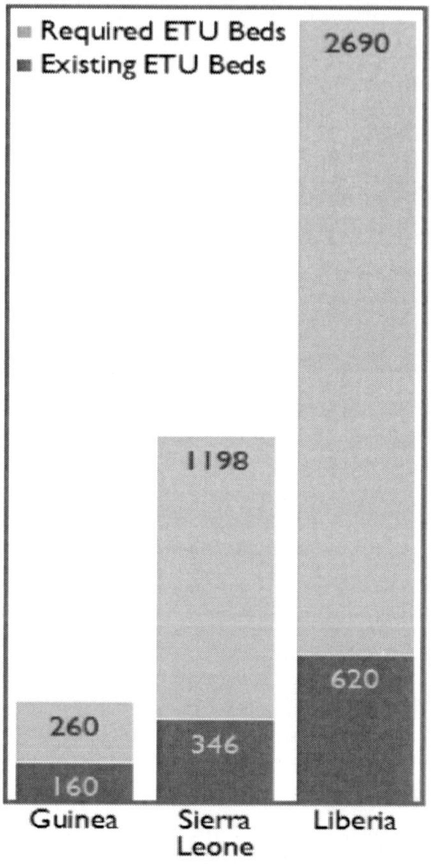


Source: Created by CRS Global Health Specialist Tiaji Salaam-Blyther from WHO, *WHO: Ebola Response Roadmap Situation Report*, October 22, 2014.

Figure 5. Bed Capacity in Ebola Treatment Units by Country, (as of October 18-19, 2014).

Safe disposal of dead bodies is also improving in Liberia, where roughly 90% of dead bodies are being removed within 24 hours of being reported to the National Call Center.[27] EVD responders are also working with community leaders to adapt traditional funeral practices that can facilitate EVD transmission, such as kissing and touching corpses.

The poor quality of health care delivery is also a concern. Inconsistent adherence to infection control protocol, for example, is contributing to EVD cases among health workers.

In July, CDC investigated a cluster of Ebola cases among HCWs in Liberia and identified "multiple opportunities for transmission of Ebola virus to HCWs, including exposure to patients with undetected Ebola in the hospital, inadequate use of personal protective equipment during cleaning and disinfection of environmental surfaces in the hospital, and potential transmission from an ill HCW to another HCW."[28] During a September tour of Liberia, CDC Director Tom Frieden noted inconsistent availability and use of gloves and hand washing.[29]

Interruptions in water supply in health clinics further hamper efforts to ensure necessary sanitation. Dr. Frieden noted of 29 health centers surveyed during his tour to the affected region, only one had running water.[30]

The poor conditions of the health facilities also discourage attendance. Power outages and interruptions in potable water delivery are common.[31] In addition, ambulance services are virtually non-existent in rural areas and limited in urban areas. One district in Sierra Leone with a population of 465,000 people reportedly has only four ambulances, which are often overcrowded with ill people, irrespective of Ebola infection status.[32]

## Commodities/Supply Chain Networks

Shortages of protective gear are associated with EVD cases among health workers, and may allow EVD to be spread within health facilities. The affected countries have limited supplies of appropriate protective equipment and not all health and support personnel who interact with the public have access to such equipment. Due to resource constraints, the protective equipment is primarily provided to healthcare workers in Ebola treatment centers, leaving health workers who operate among the general population at risk of contracting and spreading the disease (and other infectious diseases) should they encounter an undiagnosed EVD case. WHO noted, however, shortages of PPE even in ETUs.[33]

Health providers also lack sufficient supplies of antibiotics and safe blood to treat Ebola. The price of disinfectants and medicine has reportedly doubled, as people attempt to protect themselves and self-medicate in light of health system deficiencies.[34]

Transporting aid workers and commodities across and within the affected countries is complicated by poor road conditions and the suspension of air service by several commercial airlines. Efforts by the international community to develop alternative transportation routes have improved the situation, though limited air service remains a problem.

## Information

Awareness about preventing EVD infection has improved, but due to poverty, infrastructural deficiencies (e.g. clean water and sanitation), and health system constraints, many people lack means to avoid infection. Before Ebola hit, hunger was already a problem in the affected countries, particularly in rural areas.

Consumption of wild animals is common practice, particularly in areas with high food insecurity. Health officials have been expanding efforts to inform the public about the risks associated with eating wild animals, including fruit bats and other animals that might carry EVD.[35] Without sufficient access to food, hunger often compels people to continue hunting and eating the animals despite the risks.

Efforts to contain the outbreak are encumbered by weak laboratory and surveillance systems. Health experts are uncertain about how many EVD cases exist and where they are occurring, particularly in Liberia where roughly 20% of EVD cases have been confirmed through laboratory diagnosis (**Figure 6**). Limited laboratory capacity has resulted in extensive diagnosis backlogs, further calling into question the number of EVD cases and hindering efforts to contain the outbreak.

Uncertainty about EVD cases endangers health workers, other patients, and those living among people sickened by diseases of undetermined origins.

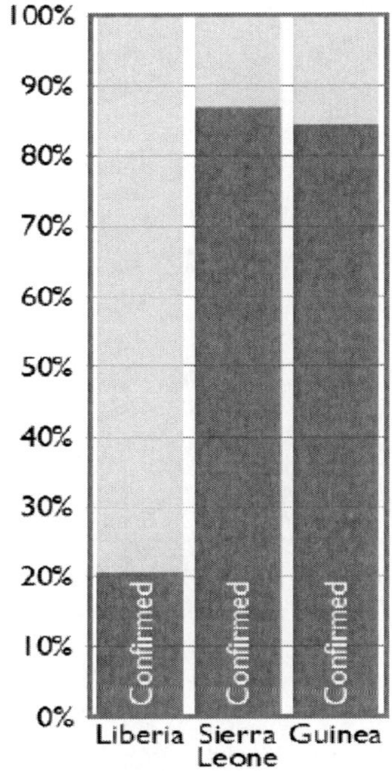


Source: Created by CRS Global Health Specialist Tiaji Salaam-Blyther from WHO, *WHO: Ebola Response Roadmap Situation Report*, October 22, 2014.

Figure 6. Laboratory Confirmed EVD Cases by Country, (as of October 22, 2014).

## INTERNATIONAL HEALTH RESPONSES

International responses are accelerating, though it remains to be seen how much it will ultimately cost to contain the outbreak and when this will be achieved. The financial requirements for containing the outbreak are rising along with the spread of the outbreak (**Figure 7**). In March, WHO estimated that it would take $4.8 million to contain the outbreak. At the end of April, more than 200 EVD cases had been discovered in Guinea, less than a dozen in Liberia, and none in Sierra Leone. In August, the organization revised its Ebola response plan, estimating it would cost roughly $490 million to contain the outbreak.[36] By then, the outbreak had reached Sierra Leone and Nigeria and had caused 3,685 EVD cases, including 1,841 deaths. The outbreak is continuing to spread, is causing broader social and economic disruptions, and has infected more than 10,000 people.

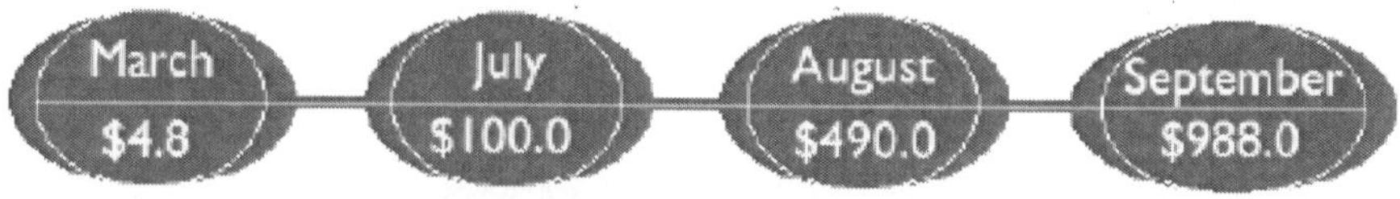


Source: Created by CRS Global Health Specialist Tiaji Salaam-Blyther from WHO and UNOCHA funding requests.

Figure 7. Timeline of International EVD Funding Requests; (U.S. millions).

**Table 3. United Nations Ebola Response Plan (U.S. $ millions)**

| | CommonServices | Guinea | Liberia | Sierra Leone | Total |
|---|---|---|---|---|---|
| **(1) Stop the Outbreak** | | | | | |
| Case identification and contact tracing | 7.0 | 26.8 | 116.5 | 39.2 | 189.5 |
| Safe and dignified burials | 0.8 | 4.3 | 14.2 | 4.4 | 23.8 |
| **(2) Treat the Infected** | | | | | |
| Ebola care and infection control | 7.0 | 52.5 | 212.6 | 59.2 | 331.2 |
| Medical care for responders | 10.0 | 1.0 | 2.0 | 1.0 | 14.0 |
| **(3) Ensure Essential Services** | | | | | |
| Food aid | 2.5 | 28.4 | 36.3 | 40.4 | 107.7 |
| Basic health care | 1.0 | 47.1 | 12.9 | 36.1 | 97.1 |
| Cash incentives for health workers | 0.0 | 2.5 | 0.0 | 0.0 | 2.5 |
| Recovery and economy | 0.3 | 9.5 | 43.1 | 11.7 | 64.8 |
| **(4) Preserve Stability** | | | | | |
| Supply chain management | 3.9 | 3.1 | 20.7 | 14.8 | 42.6 |
| Transport and fuel | 22.9 | 0.0 | 0.5 | 0.0 | 23.4 |
| Social mobilization | 0.6 | 18.6 | 13.2 | 13.3 | 45.8 |
| Messaging | 1.5 | 0.3 | 1.1 | 0.3 | 3.2 |
| Regional support for Points 1-4 | 11.9 | 0.0 | 0.0 | 0.0 | 0.0 |
| **(5) Prevent Outbreaks in Unaffected Countries** | | | | | |
| Multi-faceted/preparedness (regional) | 30.5 | 0.0 | 0.0 | 0.0 | 30.5 |
| Total | 88.0 | 194.1 | 473.1 | 220.4 | 987.8 |

Source: United Nations Office for the Coordination of Humanitarian Affairs (UNOCHA), *Ebola Virus Disease Outbreak: Overview of Needs and Requirements*, September 2014.

Notes: The amounts in the table reflect the totals indicated in the U.N. plan. Due to rounding, the subtotals do not always equal the amount indicated in the Total column.

In September, the United Nations (U.N.) established the U.N. Mission for Ebola Emergency Response (UNMEER) to coordinate the international response to the outbreak. That month, the United Nations Security Council held a special meeting on Ebola, urging member states to expedite support for the affected countries and to contribute to a U.N. integrated Ebola response plan. The six-month, $988 million plan calls for addressing the health and social impacts of the outbreak (**Table 3**).[37] Roughly half of the funds would be spent on health programs and the balance would be spent on addressing issues such as food insecurity, economic disruptions, and establishing and maintaining supply chain networks.

As of October 29, 2014, donors have contributed $493 million towards the UN plan and pledged to provide an additional $279 million (**Figure 8**).[38] Donors are also providing resources for addressing the Ebola outbreak outside of the UN response. The United Nations Office for the Coordination of Humanitarian Affairs (UNOCHA) estimates that some $894 million has been committed for addressing the outbreak and an additional $938 million has been pledged for the immediate and long-term preparedness needs. WHO and UNOCHA will likely revise their requests for funding and material support as the outbreak continues to spread.

## WHO Ebola Response Roadmap

As indicated above, roughly half of the U.N. request for tackling the outbreak is aimed at addressing direct health impacts. The World Health Organization is leading that component and has outlined measures the international community would need to take to contain the outbreak by January 2014. In the plan, entitled the Ebola Response Roadmap, WHO requested donors provide roughly $490 million for:

- building 158 referring and isolation centers capable of holding over 1,500 beds;
- increasing diagnostic capacity to process 600 samples monthly; and
- attracting more than 13,000 health workers to provide health care, conduct contact tracing, and institute safe burial protocols.

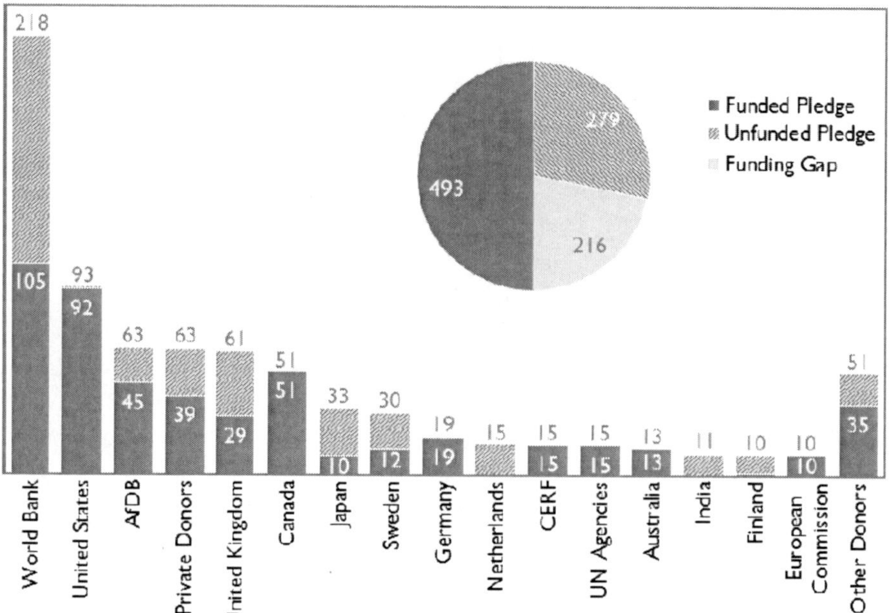


Source: Created by CRS from UNOCHA, Financial Tracking Service webpage on the Ebola outbreak at http://fts.unocha.org/, accessed on October 22, 2014.

Figure 8. Pledges, Commitments, and Disbursements for UN Ebola Plan; (as of October 27, 2014).

## WHO Community Care Campaign

Since September, pledges to send health workers to the region have increased, though human resource constraints continue to inhibit containment efforts. Since September, several countries have pledged medical support to the region, including Cuba's commitment to deploy 165 health professionals;[39] a U.S. commitment to deploy 65 U.S. Public Health Service Commissioned Corps officers for providing Ebola care in an DOD-established ETU;[40] Britain's provision of 750 troops, including medical officers;[41] and China's pledge to send more than 170 health workers.[42] The African Union and East African Community have respectively committed to send 100 and 600 health workers.[43]

In light of human resource constraints, the Liberian Government, WHO, CDC, and other partners developed the Community Care Campaign, which will initially be targeted at "the 400,000 most vulnerable households in

Liberia" and will be subsequently expanded to cover the rest of the country and region.[44] The Community Care Campaign calls for the establishment of community care centers (CCCs), which will be managed and staffed by non-governmental organizations (NGOs), community health workers (CHWs, lay people with rudimentary health training) and family members of EVD patients. The CCCs are intended to "complement" Ebola Treatment Units that are staffed by trained health practitioners and are operating at maximum capacity. The Sierra Leonean government and implementing partners are also establishing CCCS in the country. **Table 4** summarizes similarities and differences between the two facilities.

**Table 4. Similarities and Differences between ETUs and CCCs**

| | Ebola Treatment Units | Community Care Centers |
|---|---|---|
| Bed Capacity | up to 100 beds | up to 15 beds |
| EVD Diagnosis | yes | depends on facility |
| Healthcare for EVD patientsa | intravenous care, including hydration and blood transfusion; maintenance of oxygen and blood pressure levels; and treatment of other infections | oral rehydration, pain killers, fever reducers, and antimalarials |
| EVD Care | provided by trained medics | provided by NGOs, CHWs and family members |
| Oversight of Ebola Care Practices | on-site | off-site |
| Access to food and water | yes | yes |

Source: Created by CRS from WHO, Key Considerations for the Implementation of an Ebola Care Unit at Community Level, September 2014.

[a] For more on care and treatment of EVD symptoms, see http://www.cdc.gov/vhf/ebola/treatment/.

## U.S. RESPONSES TO PANDEMIC THREATS AND EBOLA

The United States is the leading funder of the international Ebola response and its financial support is continuing to rise. The U.S. Agency for International Development (USAID) reports that as of October 22, U.S.

humanitarian funding for EVD responses totaled $344.6 million.[45] In addition, the Department of Defense (DOD) is planning to spend more than $1 billion on containing the outbreak in support of U.S. EVD activities in West Africa, as described below.[46]

On October 17, President Obama established an Ebola Czar to coordinate U.S. domestic and global responses to the Ebola outbreak. The U.S. Global Ebola strategy has four key goals:

1) control the outbreak,
2) mitigate second order impacts,
3) establish coherent leadership and operations, and
4) advance global health security.

U.S. global efforts focus primarily on Liberia, where the outbreak is most widely spread, although the United States is engaged in all three affected countries. As of October 25, nearly 900 U.S. Government personnel are stationed in the region, more than 700 of which are among the 4,000 military personnel who will be deployed to the region.[47]

U.S. responses to the current Ebola outbreak are built on prior and ongoing efforts to build the capacity of foreign nations to prepare and respond to disease outbreaks—including Ebola. These activities are primarily implemented through USAID and CDC, though the U.S. Departments of Agriculture, Defense, and State also contribute to such efforts. Pandemic preparedness programs began in earnest after the 2005 avian flu outbreak and have experienced varying levels of congressional support. The section below briefly describes U.S. pandemic preparedness efforts, including Ebola outbreak responses, by agency.

## USAID Pandemic Preparedness Efforts

Since 2005, USAID has invested roughly $1 billion on helping countries detect, prepare for, and respond to outbreaks that originate in animals, such as Ebola, and that have the potential to cause pandemics. [48] In FY2014, USAID spent $72.5 million on such efforts through the Emerging and Pandemic Threats (EPT) program, which operates in 18 countries in Africa and Asia. The program grew out of USAID's initial response to H5N1 avian influenza in 2005.

Congress appropriates funds directly to USAID for EPT. These funds have fluctuated between FY2005-FY2014 (**Table 5**). Related activities in 18 countries in East and Central Africa and South and Southeast Asia focus on:

- **viral detection**—identification of viruses in wildlife, livestock, and human populations that may be public health threats;
- **risk determination**—characterization of the potential risk and method of transmission for specific viruses of animal origin;
- **institutionalization of a "one health" approach**—integration of a multi-sector approach to public health (including animal health and environment);
- **outbreak response capacity**—support for sustainable, country-level response to include preparedness and coordination; and
- **risk reduction**—promotion of actions that minimize or eliminate the potential for the emergence and spread of new viral threats.

### *USAID Ebola Responses*[49]

USAID has deployed a Disaster Assistance Response Team (DART) to West Africa to coordinate the U.S. Government's response to the Ebola outbreak. In coordination with other federal agencies, the team is overseeing the U.S. response. Between March and October 2014, USAID has committed to provide more than $300 million for combating Ebola in West Africa.[50] This included the provision of resources for 1,000 treatment beds, 130,000 sets of protective equipment for healthcare staff and outbreak investigators, as well as 50,000 hygiene kits, which include soap, bleach, gloves, masks, and other supplies to help prevent the spread of disease. [51] USAID is also supporting the International Federation of Red Cross and Red Crescent Societies (IFRC) to raise public awareness of Ebola's mode of transmission, teach disease prevention practices to communities, train volunteers to detect Ebola symptoms and identify contacts of confirmed or suspected cases for further monitoring, and support safe burial and body management activities. USAID has reprogrammed funds from the Global Heath and International Disaster Assistance accounts to fund these efforts.

**Table 5. USAID Pandemic Preparedness Funding (current U.S. $ millions and percent)**

| | FY05 Actual | FY06 Actual | FY07 Actual | FY08 Actual | FY09 Actual | FY10 Actual | FY11 Actual | FY12 Actual | FY13 Actual | FY14 Estimate | FY15 Request | FY14-FY15 |
|---|---|---|---|---|---|---|---|---|---|---|---|---|
| Avian Flu/ Pandemic Preparedness | 16 | 162 | 161 | 115 | 190 | 106 | 93 | 58 | 55 | 73 | 50 | -31.0% |

Source: Created by CRS correspondence with USAID officials, August 6, 2014.

Note: Includes supplemental appropriations.

**Table 6. CDC Global Disease Detection Funding (current U.S. $ millions)**

| | FY04 Actual | FY05 Actual | FY06 Actual | FY07 Actual | FY08 Actual | FY09 Actual | FY10 Actual | FY11 Actual | FY12 Actual | FY13 Actual | FY14 Estimate | FY15 Estimate |
|---|---|---|---|---|---|---|---|---|---|---|---|---|
| GDD | 12 | 21 | 32 | 32 | 31 | 34 | 44 | 42 | 42 | 45 | 45 | 45 |

Source: Created by CRS from correspondence with the Office of Management and Budget (OMB), appropriations legislation, and budget justification documents.

## CDC Pandemic Preparedness Efforts

CDC funds its global pandemic preparedness efforts through a variety of accounts, including the Global Disease Detection (GDD) program, Emerging and Zoonotic Infectious Diseases, Global Health, Immunization and Respiratory Diseases, and Public Health Preparedness and Response. The Centers leverage resources from these and other program accounts to respond to global disease outbreaks—including Ebola. Appropriations for GDD have grown since 2003 (**Table 6**).

CDC has requested additional support ($45 million) in FY2015 to fund activities in support of the Global Health Security Agenda, which will accelerate activities to detect, prevent, and respond to global infectious disease threats like Ebola.[52] CDC directly or indirectly supports pandemic influenza preparedness efforts in more than 50 countries. In some cases, CDC sends experts to work with WHO country offices or foreign health ministries, and at other times, CDC forms cooperative agreements with partners to support country efforts.

### *CDC Ebola Responses*[53]

At the end of March 2014, CDC teams traveled to Guinea and Liberia to help those Health Ministries characterize and control the outbreak, identify and manage EVD cases, conduct contact tracing, and improve data management. Following an initial response, new cases flared up after appearing to decelerate for some time. CDC returned to the region and began resumed technical assistance efforts. In addition to the activities discussed above, CDC is also training airport personnel and working with partners to display Ebola-specific travel messages for electronic monitors and posters at airports in the affected countries. CDC is not providing direct care of Ebola patients. As of October 22, 2014, CDC has committed more than $16.7 million for its Ebola responses.[54]

## Department of Defense Ebola Responses

Until recently, DOD responses to the outbreak were focused on researching treatments and vaccines and providing laboratory diagnostic assistance to Sierra Leone and Liberia. On September 8, DOD announced that it would provide $22 million to set up a 25-bed field hospital in Liberia that would be used to treat EVD cases among healthcare workers. The Department of Health and Human Services (HHS) U.S. Public Health Service Commissioned Corps will deploy 65 officers "to Liberia to manage and staff the hospital."[55] Military personnel will establish and supply the facility, but not provide direct medical care.[56]

On September 16, President Barack Obama announced the launch of "Operation United Assistance."[57] The operation is to be based in Monrovia, Liberia, will entail the deployment of roughly 4,000 U.S. military forces, and be overseen and coordinated by the DOD U.S. Africa Command. The operation will support:

- the coordination of U.S. and international relief efforts;
- the provision of medical personnel to train up to 200 health workers weekly; and
- the establishment of 12 treatment centers in Liberia, each with 100-bed capacity.

Operation-related efforts are underway. The first 22-bed ETC is expected to be completed by the end of October and three others are to be completed in November.[58] More than 700 U.S. military personnel are in the region, including personnel from the U.S. Naval Medical Research Center who are operating three mobile medical labs for EVD testing.[59] Congress has approved several DOD reprogramming requests to fund Operation United Assistance as well as other related activities, including those that supply personal protective equipment, laboratory inputs, and technical advisors to the region. Total DOD funding for the global Ebola response is expected to exceed $1 billion.[60]

## POSSIBLE ISSUES FOR CONGRESS

The current Ebola outbreak has overwhelmed the governments of Guinea, Sierra Leone, and Liberia. Insufficient capacity to detect, treat, and prevent the spread of disease has enabled the virus to spread and has further weakened health systems that were already inundated and in dilapidated conditions. Congress has held several hearings on the outbreak and enacted legislation that urged expanding U.S. and international responses and that provided funds for U.S. responses. As the outbreak continues to spread, the Administration may request additional funds to contain the outbreak. This section describes issues Congress may consider as it assesses U.S. and international responses.

## Human Resource Constraints

At the end of August, WHO estimated that it would take 13,000 health workers to contain the Ebola outbreak.[61] Although foreign governments and non-governmental organizations are beginning to deploy medics and other health workers, their numbers are not sufficient to meet the human resource demands. Human resource constraints are most acute in Liberia, where access to Ebola care is the most limited. The United States has partnered with the Liberian government, WHO, and other groups to develop a Community Care Campaign (see "WHO Community Care Campaign"). Doctors Without Borders (known by its French acronym, MSF) has expressed concern about the Community Care Campaign, asserting that the CCCs could turn into "contamination centers" without strict infection control, adequate supplies, trained staff, regular supervision, the ability to diagnose and refer patients, and proper burial methods.[62] WHO acknowledges that "any deficiencies in the quality of implementation could present major risk of virus transmission within the CCC thus exacerbating a situation it is set out to address."[63] Key factors that may complicate safe implementation of the Community Care Campaign include:

- **Quality control.** Inconsistent adherence to infection control protocol is reportedly contributing to EVD cases among health workers. The inability to ensure disease infection, prevention, and control (IPC) protocols among trained health personnel calls into question whether non-governmental organizations, community health workers, and family members will adhere to IPC protocols. This concern is particularly acute for lay personnel (like family members) who may provide Ebola care in the CCCs.
- **Family care providers.** To avoid the possible spread of EVD from familial caretakers to other community members, WHO recommends that only one family member provide care for each patient for the duration of their stay in the CCCs. WHO specifies that the "family member providing supportive care to the patient must not go back and forth between the CCC and the community."[64] However, collective familial care of and close community interaction with the ill is common in Liberia. It is unclear whether CCC supervisors will be able to curtail this custom and ensure that only one family member provides care. Other factors, including loss of income, separation of the caretaker from their uninfected family members, or emotional

stress from being in a CCC, might also discourage compliance with WHO familial care guidelines.

- **Waste management and safe burial practices.** IPC protocol requires that those handling the soiled linen of EVD patients, cleaning the CCCs, or burying victims of EVD wear personal protective equipment (PPE). Further, in order to prevent the spread of EVD within CCCs, caretakers must follow strict protocol in using PPE and managing waste (using only designated areas for waste disposal and ensuring daily collection of human and PPE waste). The affected countries face deficiencies in waste management. In 2012, less than 20% of people living in the affected countries had access to improved sanitation facilities.[65] It may be a challenge ensuring strict adherence to IPC protocol among lay care takers without medical training, particularly if they lack access to sanitation themselves.
- **Oversight.** According to WHO, "monitoring and supervision is critical in ensuring the success of the approach."[66] Most of the "low level community health workers and members of the community" who will be tasked with providing care in CCCs have never done so before. The Community Care Campaign calls for once daily supervisory visits by at least one health care worker trained in IPC. It remains to be seen whether once daily visits are enough to ensure compliance with the IPC protocols, as well as others, including proper and consistent use of PPE by care takers, launderers, burial team, and sanitation workers.
- **Supply chain management.** Due to poor supply chain management practices, many publicly funded health clinics in the affected countries face interruptions in medical supplies and often lack commodities such as gloves, masks, and gowns. A lack of protective equipment in ETUs and health clinics has been associated with EVD infection among health workers.[67] Lapses in protective gear in CCCs can lead to unsafe practices, such as recycling or reusing existing PPE. It remains to be seen whether WHO and its partners will be able to ensure the continuous supply of commodities to disparate CCCs.

WHO recognizes the inherent risks of this effort and advises that Ministries of Health in the affected countries "embark on this approach in an incremental manner starting with a few pilots that are well monitored before taking it up to scale."[68]

U.S. implementation of the Community Care Campaign is already underway. USAID is issuing grants to non-governmental organizations to oversee the management of Community Care Centers. The White House reports that the United States Government has already provided 9,000 community care kits in Liberia for use by individuals in their homes.[69] NGOs generally have autonomy over the implementation of USAID grants, and USAID oversees implementation to ensure that program targets are met. Questions abound, however, about U.S. oversight and implementation of this campaign, particularly regarding U.S. government oversight of grantees managing CCCs and the standardization of quality control and IPC protocol.

## Leadership of the International Outbreak Response

Observers have criticized WHO leadership over the global Ebola response. Some critics have contended that budget cuts that began under WHO's reform efforts have made the Organization less effective and have limited its capacity to contain the outbreak.[70] The 2014-2015 WHO program budget called for a 51% reduction in outbreak and crisis response activities from 2012-2013 levels.[71] Some observers maintain that earlier budget cuts have also crippled the agency by reducing critical staff, causing the closure of the viral hemorrhagic fever unit, and undermining operational capacity.[72] Beyond budgetary constraints, some critics contended that WHO's response has been stymied by bureaucratic bloat and undue influence of underqualified staff who attained their positions due to political relationships.[73]

Weak health systems in the affected countries, inadequate capacity of WHO to carry out its own Ebola plans, as well as insufficient international responses to the outbreak have reignited debates about whether WHO should function primarily as an advisory body or maintain some form of operational capacity. Some analysts advocate for the establishment of a WHO-administered "Health Systems Fund," that could be used to both build long-term health system capacity, as well as address short-term crises like the ongoing Ebola outbreak.[74] While supporting the need for a ready-to-deploy team of emergency health responders, others assert the "politics of sovereignty" would preclude WHO from leading such an effort.[75]

## U.S. Support for Ebola Responses and Health Systems

The speed at which EVD is spreading across West Africa is attributable, in large part, to weak health systems in those countries. Donors have long grappled with how to address health emergencies in light of dysfunctional health systems. In the early 2000s, donors turned to disease-based funding and channeled health aid through non-governmental groups. Opponents of this approach argued that disease-specific programs exacerbate human resource shortages in the public sector and further weaken health systems when parallel bureaucracies are established and government authorities are bypassed. Supporters assert that disease-based funding strengthens oversight capacity and facilitates the monitoring and evaluation of the investments.

This debate intensified following the introduction of the President's Emergency Plan for AIDS Relief (PEPFAR).[76] In an effort to curb the massive number of deaths that followed the introduction of HIV/AIDS, U.S. agencies provided funding to large non-governmental organizations and local partners who established care and treatment facilities outside of government networks. While the effort helped save millions of lives and averted millions more HIV infections, the United States became the sole supporter for millions of people worldwide whose lives would be at risk should U.S. funding be discontinued. In the second phase of PEPFAR (FY2009-FY2013), increasing portions of PEPFAR resources were used to support health systems in hopes of bolstering country capacity to assume ownership over HIV/AIDS programs. Now in its third phase, debate on the use of PEPFAR funds for building health systems has resumed. A 2013 GAO report noted that roughly 21% of PEPFAR funds were spent on capacity building projects under the "other" budgetary category. At her confirmation hearing, PEPFAR Country Coordinator Deborah Birx asserted that under her leadership, 50% of all PEPFAR resources, including those funded through other accounts, would be spent on care and treatment activities, as mandated. Health system advocates fear that budgetary reforms aimed at adhering to the law may imperil efforts to bolster health systems.

The U.S. Congress faces a similar dilemma with the current Ebola outbreak. The affected countries need focused support to contain and end this outbreak. If and when the outbreak is arrested, however, the countries may not be in any better position to detect, prevent, or respond to other potential disease outbreaks unless donors begin the arduous task of supporting the development of strong health systems. Ken Isaacs, Vice President of International Programs and Government Relations at Samaritan's Purse, described this dilemma at an August 2014 congressional hearing on Ebola, stating "While it should be the goal of the developed world to build capacity, the building of this capacity should not be the focus during times of an emergency crisis of a deadly disease that threatens the international community."[77] USAID has reportedly established an Ebola Health Systems Strengthening working group to support the resumption of health care delivery and to bolster the health systems once the outbreak is contained.[78]

Though PEPFAR and other U.S.-funded health programs have attempted to respond to calls for greater investment in health systems, no appropriations specifically targeting such efforts are provided. Language in appropriations and accompanying conference reports direct the majority of health aid to particular diseases, leaving minimal resources for broader activities to strengthen health systems. The inability of the affected countries to respond to an unforeseen health event may prompt Congress to review how global health funds are appropriated.

## Evaluating U.S. Responses

A variety of U.S. agencies are responding to the ongoing Ebola outbreak. The Department of State is leading diplomatic engagements; USAID is coordinating U.S. responses, including the provision of financial and material support; CDC is heading public health and medical response activities; and DOD is handling support for foreign armed forces. With the exception of USAID, the budgetary structure of each of these agencies enables them to respond to this unanticipated event by drawing from accounts that have flexible authorities. The Department of State's efforts to coordinate bilateral diplomatic engagements are conducted through existing channels (e.g., embassy contacts) and, as such, would not require additional, dedicated funding. Outbreak responses by the CDC can be financed through USAID disaster assistance accounts, as well as several CDC accounts that are used for domestic and international health efforts and for which there is not explicit congressional direction on their use. The DOD budget also supports an array of domestic and international health activities that do not receive detailed congressional direction.

Congress has established numerous directives over the years on how foreign aid funds are to be used. As the lead U.S. development agency, USAID often receives specific direction from Congress on how the bulk of its funds will be used through annual appropriations, leaving the agency with limited ability to address unanticipated events, like the current Ebola outbreak, without drawing from ongoing health efforts. According to USAID, it is currently reprogramming funds planned for preventing future outbreaks, as well as addressing ongoing outbreaks (including responses to H7N9 avian influenza in China and MERS-CoV in the Middle East), to address the current Ebola outbreak.[79]

Supporters of the current appropriation structure see it as a tool for overseeing health programs and ensuring that congressional priorities are met. Opponents argue that congressional directives encumber the agility that is needed in the field and create artificial segmentation of health and development issues, thereby limiting the impact and sustainability of such efforts.

By their nature, disease outbreaks are often unpredictable, though with appropriate disease surveillance, detection, and response mechanisms, their impact can be minimized. At present, USAID pandemic preparedness efforts are focused on East and Central Africa, where previous Ebola and influenza outbreaks have occurred, as well as South and Southeast Asia. Now that Ebola has emerged in West Africa, another EVD outbreak may occur in the region; a scenario the affected countries may be ill-prepared to handle. The FY2015 budget request ($50 million) for pandemic preparedness is roughly 30% less than the FY2014 funding level ($73 million). Even if Congress funds USAID pandemic preparedness programs at the FY2014 funding level, one USAID official contends that it will not be enough to meet current demands.[80]

## Addressing the Long-Term and Broader Effects of the Outbreak

Under the best of circumstances, experts predict that the outbreak can be contained by the end of January. In the meantime, the high death tolls are disrupting social structures and may cause broad, long-term effects in the region. MSF has reported that some affected villages in Sierra Leone have lost the majority of adult community members, leaving vulnerable populations—such as children and the elderly—without resources to cultivate agricultural land and procure food.[81] Observers are also concerned about a growing number of children who are being orphaned from Ebola. This group is particularly vulnerable to marginalization due to overwhelming fear of the virus. Countries in West and Central Africa already had large orphan populations due to a variety of causes including armed conflict and HIV/AIDS. In 2012, some 28 million children were orphaned in the region, of whom more than 4 million lost one or more parent to AIDS.[82] The outbreak is also hindering the capacity of these governments to address other health issues, such as obstetrical complications. Experts are concerned that child and maternal mortality rates, already high in the region, may further rise due to diminishing numbers of health personnel (caused both by Ebola deaths and abandonment of posts), diversion of limited resources to Ebola treatment centers, and public avoidance of health centers.

The full health effects of the Ebola outbreak may not be known until it is contained. An accounting of broader health and development needs will likely ensue and may rekindle debate over how U.S. global health assistance funds are apportioned. Congress is likely to face arguments from advocates from a variety of actors attempting to garner support for a bevy of health and development issues that will have likely worsened in the wake of Ebola, including maternal and child mortality, child vulnerability and orphanhood, poverty, food scarcity, and water-borne infections.

## Considering Research and Development Needs

Since 1976, several Ebola outbreaks have erupted in sub-Saharan Africa, yet therapeutic options remain undeveloped. There is no specific cure, treatment, or vaccine for Ebola, nor or is there any post-exposure prophylaxis for health workers who face regular exposure. Treatment of EVD symptoms increases the probability of survival. Several experimental specific treatments and vaccines are beginning clinical trials to determine their safety and efficacy. The appropriate use of experimental drugs that have not been tested for human safety and effectiveness has become a matter of debate, particularly around the issue of equity.

A global health lawyer described the ensuing debate. "Should [U.S.] workers receive a drug in extremely scarce supply when Africans are affected in far greater numbers? Balanced against this sense of injustice is the ethical concern of administering an experimental drug to African patients that has not undergone any safety testing in humans."[83] In addition, if the experimental drugs are ineffectual or cause serious side effects, then their use may further exacerbate mistrust in healthcare workers and modern medical treatments. WHO held a special meeting in August on the topic and announced that under "the particular circumstances of th[e] outbreak, and provided certain conditions are met ... it is ethical to offer unproven interventions with as yet unknown efficacy and adverse effects, as potential treatment or prevention."[84]

In October, press reports indicated that WHO planned to begin testing two Ebola vaccines in January on some 20,000 health workers and other volunteers. The organization also indicated that a limited amount of an experimental treatment might be available for use in Liberia by early November.[85] At the end of October, WHO convened a meeting "with high-ranking government representatives from Ebola-affected countries and development partners, civil society, regulatory agencies, vaccine manufacturers and funding agencies yesterday to discuss and agree on how to fast track testing and deployment of vaccines in sufficient numbers to impact the Ebola epidemic."[86] Once the trials commence, debates about ethical practices will likely ensue, particularly if trial participants die or experience other adverse reactions.

## CONCLUSION

In an August 29, 2014 report, WHO warned that bordering countries, namely Benin, Burkina Faso, Côte d'Ivoire, Guinea-Bissau, Mali, and Senegal, were "at risk" of seeing Ebola cases.[87] On October 23, 2014, Mali reported its first Ebola case and health officials suspect that cases may exist in other neighboring countries. WHO is reportedly helping neighboring countries to build EVD surveillance, preparedness and response plans. An Oxford University study concluded that some 22 million people across Central and West Africa live in forested areas where one of the suspected vectors (fruit bats) resides,[88] raising concerns among some that future Ebola outbreaks may occur in the region and other parts of sub-Saharan Africa. The article notes that "changes in human mobility and connectivity will likely have profound impacts on the dispersion of Ebola cases." Prospects for future Ebola outbreaks in urban areas and in countries with limited pandemic preparedness capacity raise several questions, including:

- Is the U.S. response to the Ebola outbreak effective?
- Does the United Stated sufficiently support pandemic preparedness efforts?
- Does disease-specific funding encumber pandemic preparedness efforts?
- Will the reprogramming of USAID funds to address the Ebola outbreak impact ongoing global health and development programs?

- Are ongoing outbreak responses by the U.S. and international improving the capacity of the affected countries, as well as others in the region, to identify, detect, and respond to future outbreaks?

## End Notes

[1] This section was summarized from WHO, *Ebola*, fact sheet, number 103, April 2014.

[2] WHO, "WHO: Air travel is low-risk for Ebola transmission," Note for the Media, August 14, 2014 and WHO, "Statement on travel and transport in relation to Ebola virus disease (EVD) outbreak, August 18, 2014.

[3] "WHO urges calm as Kenya bans contact with Ebola-affected countries," *The Guardian*, August 17, 2014.

[4] WHO, *Situation Report Update*, September 8, 2014.

[5] Abby Ohlheiser, "WHO sending experts to Mali after first Ebola diagnosis in the West African country," *Washington Post,* October 24, 2014.

[6] The Guardian, "WHO aims for Ebola serum in weeks and vaccine tests in Africa by January," September 22, 2014.

[7] WHO, *Interim Infection Prevention and Control Guidance for Care of Patients with Suspected or Confirmed Filovirus Haemorrhagic Fever in Health-Care Settings, with Focus on Ebola*, August 2014.

[8] Martin Meltzer et al., "Estimating the Future Number of Cases in the Ebola Epidemic—Liberia and Sierra Leone, 2014-2015," *MMWR*, (September 23, 2014), volume 63.

[9] This section was summarized by CRS from WHO, *Ebola virus disease – Democratic Republic of Congo*, Disease Outbreak News, August 27, 2014 and September 10, 2014.

[10] WHO, *Ebola Response Roadmap Situation Report*, October 22, 2014.

[11] H.Res. 701, Expressing the sense of the House of Representatives that the current outbreak of Ebola in Guinea, Sierra Leone, and Liberia is an international health crisis and is the largest and most widespread outbreak of the disease ever recorded and S.Res. 541, Recognizing the severe threat that the Ebola outbreak in West Africa poses to populations, governments, and economies across Africa and, if not properly contained, to regions across the globe, and expressing support for those affected by this epidemic.

[12] For more information on health systems, see http://www.who.int/topics/health_systems/en/.

[13] Naina Bajekal, "Ebola Lockdown in Sierra Leone Finds 150 New Cases," *Time*, September 22, 2014 and Umaru Fofana, "Sierra Leone wraps up three-day Ebola lockdown," *Reuters*, September 21, 2014.

[14] USAID, *West Africa Ebola Outbreak—Update #2*, August 11, 2014.

[15] United Nations Office for the Coordination of Humanitarian Affairs (UNOCHA), *Ebola Virus Disease Outbreak: Overview of Needs and Requirements*, September 2014.

[16] UNICEF, *Trends in Maternal Mortality: 1990 to 2013*, 2014.

[17] WHO, *World Health Statistics Report*, 2014.

[18] United Nations, "Secretary-General's Remarks to the Security Council on Ebola," Press Statement, September 18, 2014.

[19] WHO, *Unprecedented number of medical staff infected with Ebola*, August 25, 2014.

[20] U.S. Congress, House Committee on Foreign Affairs, Subcommittee on Africa, Global Health, Global Human Rights and International Organizations, *Combating the Ebola Threat*, Testimony by Dr. Frank Glover, August 7, 2014.

[21] WHO, *WHO: Ebola Response Roadmap Situation Report*, October 22, 2014.

[22] WHO, "WHO Director-General briefs Geneva UN missions on the Ebola outbreak," Briefing to United Nations Member States, August 12, 2014.

[23] WHO, *Ebola Response Roadmap*, August 28, 2014, p. 24.

[24] Teleconference with CDC Director Tom Frieden, September 5, 2014.

[25] Communication with USAID, October 26, 2014.

[26] Sheri Fink, "In Liberia, a Good or Very Bad Sign: Empty Hospital Beds," *New York Times*, October 28, 2014.

[27] U.S. Government Inter-Agency Conference Call on Ebola, October 17, 2014.

[28] Joseph Forrester et al., "Cluster of Ebola Cases Among Liberian and U.S. Health Care Workers in an Ebola Treatment Unit and Adjacent Hospital – Liberia, 2014," *Morbidity and Mortality Weekly Report*, (October 17, 2014), volume 63, number 41.

[29] Teleconference with CDC Director Tom Frieden, September 5, 2014.

[30] Ibid.

[31] Doctors Without Borders, "Flash Quote: WHO Declares Ebola an International Public Health Emergency," Field News, August 8, 2014.

[32] The Star, "In Sierra Leone, an exhausting struggle to contain Ebola," August 18, 2014.

[33] WHO, "Unprecedented number of medical staff infected with Ebola," Situation Assessment, August 25, 2014.

[34] Newsweek, "Ebola Frontline: Flooding in Sierra Leone Exacerbates Public Health Fears," August 12, 2014.

[35] "Ebola risk unheeded as Guinea's villagers keep on eating fruit bats," *The Guardian*, August 4, 2014.

[36] WHO, *Ebola Response Roadmap*, August 28, 2014.

[37] United Nations Office for the Coordination of Humanitarian Affairs (UNOCHA), *Ebola Virus Disease Outbreak: Overview of Needs and Requirements*, September 2014.

[38] UNOCHA webpage on Ebola Outbreak Funding at http://fts.unocha.org, accessed on October 22, 2014.

[39] WHO, "Cuban medical team heading for Sierra Leone," Press Release, September 2014.

[40] HHS, "U.S. Public Health Service Commissioned Corps to help treat Ebola patients in Liberia," September 16, 2014.

[41] USAID, "West Africa-Ebola Outbreak," Fact Sheet #4, October 22, 2014.

[42] Ewan MacAskill and Rowena Mason, "British troops to be sent to help fight Ebola," *The Guardian*, October 8, 2014.

[43] USAID, "West Africa-Ebola Outbreak," Fact Sheet #4, October 22, 2014.

[44] White House, "Fact Sheet: U.S. Response to the Ebola Epidemic in West Africa," September 16, 2014.

[45] USAID, "West Africa-Ebola Outbreak," Fact Sheet #4, October 22, 2014.

[46] White House webpage on the U.S. Ebola response at http://www.whitehouse.gov/ebola-response, accessed on October 23, 2014.

[47] Communication with USAID, October 26, 2014.

[48] See the USAID webpage on pandemics at http://www.usaid.gov/what-we-do/global-health/

[49] Summarized from USAID, "USAID and CDC Announce Additional Assistance for West Africa Ebola Response," press release, August 5, 2014.

[50] USAID, "West Africa-Ebola Outbreak," Fact Sheet #4, October 22, 2014.

[51] U.S. Embassy, "U.S. to Help Mobilize More Health Workers for Ebola Outbreak," September 9, 2014.

[52] For more on the Global Health Security Agenda, see http://www.cdc.gov/globalhealth /security/.

[53] This section was summarized from correspondence with CDC. Also see, Meredith Dixon and Ilana Schafer, "Ebola Viral Disease Outbreak – West Africa, 2014," *Morbidity and Mortality Weekly Report* (June 27, 2014), volume 63, issue 25, pp. 548-551; and http://www.cdc.gov/vhf/ebola/outbreaks/guinea/.

[54] USAID, "West Africa-Ebola Outbreak," Fact Sheet #4, October 22, 2014.

[55] HHS, "U.S. Public Health Service Commissioned Corps to help treat Ebola patients in Liberia," Press Release, September 16, 2014.

[56] Richard Sisk, "Pentagon to Set Up Ebola Field Hospital in Liberia," Military.com, September 8, 2014; and AFP, "US to Send Field Hospital to Ebola-Hit Liberia," September 8, 2014.

[57] White House, "Fact Sheet: U.S. Response to the Ebola Epidemic in West Africa," September 16, 2014.

[58] White House, "Fact Sheet: The U.S. Government's Response to Ebola at Home and Abroad," October 22, 2014.

[59] Ibid.

[60] White House, "Fact Sheet: U.S. Response to the Ebola Epidemic in West Africa," October 6, 2014.

[61] WHO, *Ebola Response Roadmap*, August 28, 2014, p. 24.

[62] Lenny Bernstein and Lena Sun, "New effort to fight Ebola in Liberia would move infected patients out of their homes," *Washington Post*, September 22, 2014.

[63] WHO, *Key Considerations for the Implementation of an Ebola Care Unit at Community Level*, September 2014.

[64] Ibid.

[65] World Bank database, accessed on October 1, 2014.

[66] WHO, *Key Considerations for the Implementation of an Ebola Care Unit at Community Level*, September 2014.

[67] For more on health infrastructure deficiencies, see Joseph Forrester et al., "Assessment of Ebola Virus Disease, Health Care Infrastructure, and Preparedness-Four Counties, Southeastern Liberia, August 2014, *Morbidity and Mortality Weekly Report*, October 7, 2014, volume 1, issue 3.

[68] WHO, *Key Considerations for the Implementation of an Ebola Care Unit at Community Level*, September 2014.

[69] White House, "Fact Sheet: The U.S. Government's Response to Ebola at Home and Abroad," October 6, 2014.

[70] Sheri Pink, "Cuts at WHO Hurt Response to Ebola Crisis," *New York Times*, September 3, 2014.

[71] WHO, *Proposed Programme Budget 2014-2015*, April 19, 2013, Sixty-Sixth World Health Assembly, A66/7.

[72] Doctors Without Borders, "Ebola: the failures of the international outbreak response," September 2, 2014. Stehpanie Nebehay and Barbara Lewis, "WHO slashes budget, jobs in new era of austerity," *Reuters*, May 19, 2011.

[73] Jason Gale and John Lauerman, "How the World's Top Health Body Allowed Ebola to Spiral Out of Control," *Bloomberg*, October 17, 2014; Lena Sun et al., "Out of Control: How the world's health organization failed to stop the Ebola disaster," *The Washington Post*,

October 4, 2014; and Associated Press, "World Health Organization admits botching attempts to stop Ebola in West Africa," October 17, 2014.

[74] Lawrence Gostin, "West Africa's Ebola Epidemic is Out of Control, But Never Had to Happen," Briefing Paper Number 9, August 20, 2014. For more on the possible structure and functions of the Global Health Fund, see Lawrence Gostin and Eric Friedman, "Towards a Framework Convention on Global Health: A Transformative Agenda for Global Health Justice," *Yale Journal of Health Policy, Law, and Ethics*, (2013), volume 13, issue 1.

[75] Jack Chow, "The Ultimate Ebola-Fighting Force," *Foreign Policy*, September 10, 2014.

[76] For more on PEPFAR, see CRS Report IF00042, The President's Emergency Plan for AIDS Relief (PEPFAR): Summary of Recent Developments (In Focus) and CRS Report R42776, *The President's Emergency Plan for AIDS Relief (PEPFAR): Funding Issues After a Decade of Implementation, FY2004-FY2013*, by Tiaji Salaam-Blyther

[77] U.S. Congress, House Committee on Foreign Affairs, Subcommittee on Africa, Global Health, Global Human Rights and International Organizations, *Combating the Ebola Threat*, Testimony by Ken Isaacs, Vice President of International Programs and Government Relations, Samaritan's Purse, August 7, 2014

[78] USAID, *Investing in Health Systems to Address the Ebola Outbreak*, September 30, 2014.

[79] CRS correspondence with USAID, August 5, 2014.

[80] Ibid.

[81] USAID, *West Africa Ebola Outbreak—Update # 5*, August 18, 2014.

[82] UNICEF, *Towards an AIDS-Free Generation Children and AIDS: Sixth Stocktaking Report*, 2013.

[83] Lawrence Gostin et al., "The Ebola Epidemic: A Global Health Emergency," *JAMA*, (August 11, 2014).

[84] WHO, "Ethical considerations for use of unregistered interventions for Ebola viral disease (EVD)," WHO statement, August 12, 2014.

[85] The Guardian, "WHO aims for Ebola serum in weeks and vaccine tests in Africa by January," September 22, 2014.

[86] WHO, "WHO convenes industry leaders and key partners to discuss trials and production of Ebola vaccine," news release, October 24, 2014.

[87] WHO, *WHO: Ebola Response Roadmap Situation Report 1*, August 29, 2014.

[88] David Pigott et al., "Mapping the zoonotic niche of Ebola virus disease in Africa," *Elife*, (September 7, 2014).

In: Ebola
Editor: MaryAnn Cole

ISBN: 978-1-63482-253-4


*Chapter 3*

# PREVENTING THE INTRODUCTION AND SPREAD OF EBOLA IN THE UNITED STATES: FREQUENTLY ASKED QUESTIONS*

***Sarah A. Lister***

Throughout 2014, an outbreak of Ebola virus disease (EVD) has outpaced the efforts of health workers trying to contain it in three West African countries: Guinea, Liberia, and Sierra Leone. (These are often referred to as "affected countries" or "countries with widespread transmission." In mid-November, 2014, Ebola transmission also occurred for the second time in neighboring Mali. The extent of spread in Mali remains to be seen.) EVD cases have been imported to other countries, including the United States, where two nurses were infected while caring for a patient who had traveled from Liberia.

Members of Congress and the public have considered ways to prevent the entry and spread of EVD in the United States. Official recommendations have seemed to conflict at times. In part this reflects the evolution of officials' understanding of this new threat and the scientific and technical aspects of its control. In addition, under the nation's federalist governance structure, the federal and state governments are empowered to take measures to control

* This is an edited, reformatted and augmented version of a Congressional Research Service publication R43809, prepared for Members and Committees of Congress, dated December 5, 2014.

should consist of, at a minimum, a questionnaire, a temperature measurement and, if there is a fever, an assessment of the risk that the fever is caused by EVD."[23] It recommends prohibiting persons who have "an illness consistent with EVD" from departing countries with Ebola transmission unless they are undergoing medical evacuation on specially equipped air ambulances.[24]

Most land borders between Guinea, Liberia, and Sierra Leone have been formally closed by authorities, but unregulated, ad hoc cross-border traffic remains common. The main international airports in the affected countries—one in each country—remain open. The governments of the affected countries are screening departing travelers for possible Ebola infection or exposure at airports that remain open, as recommended by WHO.[25] The Centers for Disease Control and Prevention (CDC) has trained these airport personnel to undertake such screening using CDC-developed guidelines.[26] The screening being carried out is similar to the entry screening of travelers from EVD-affected countries now being undertaken by U.S. officials, and involves taking the traveler's temperature and administering a questionnaire. According to CDC, travelers may continue traveling if

- all answers to questions about EVD symptoms or exposure are "no";
- they do not show any signs or report any symptoms of EVD; and
- they do not have a fever of (or higher than) 38.6° C or 101.5° F.[27]

Travelers who exhibit signs or report symptoms consistent with EVD undergo a more thorough health screening. The United States Agency for International Development (USAID) has provided hands-free temperature scanners to the affected countries.[28] The French government and the International Committee of the Red Cross are also helping the Guinean government to improve exit screening procedures.[29]

### *Do Exit Screenings Effectively Detect EVD Cases?*

For several reasons, exit screening may not detect all current or incubating cases of Ebola virus infection. There are, by definition, no symptoms of EVD during the incubation period of the disease, which can last up to 21 days.[30] Diagnostic tests for EVD do not detect the disease during the incubation period, and may also fail to detect the infection for the first few days of symptoms.[31] Consequently, testing is not a reliable means of ruling out infection. Potential exposure, without symptoms, can only be assessed by querying the traveler. Some travelers may not disclose possible exposure due to lack of knowledge of it, or mendacity.

A group of researchers developed a mathematical model to study the effects of exit and entry screening (see "How does entry screening in the United States work?") on detection of EVD among travelers.[32] Acknowledging that neither approach (alone or together) would identify all incubating cases of illness, the authors report that the model showed exit screening to be the more effective and efficient of the two interventions, and note that many developing countries lack the capacity to conduct entry screening. However, they also comment that exit screening occurs in countries already struggling with widespread EVD transmission, so that international assistance with exit screening can assure its optimal effectiveness.

### *Does WHO Recommend Restricting Travel from Ebola-Affected Countries?*

WHO "does not recommend travel restrictions to or from the countries affected [by Ebola], except for EVD patients, contacts of EVD patients and corpses of EVD patients."[33] Its rationale is stated most recently by its Ebola Travel and Transport Task Force, which says

> Such measures can create a false impression of control and may have a detrimental impact on the number of health care workers volunteering to assist Ebola control or prevention efforts in the affected countries. Such measures may also adversely reduce essential trade, including supplies of food, fuel and medical equipment to the affected countries, contributing to their humanitarian and economic hardship.[34]

## U.S. Laws and Procedures Involving Airlines and Other Conveyances

### *How Might People Travel from Affected Countries to the United States?*[35]

There are currently no scheduled non-stop flights on commercial airlines between Guinea, Liberia, or Sierra Leone and the United States.[36] It appears that the majority of air travelers from West Africa to the United States fly via Europe.[37] As of October 2014, most flights out of the affected countries are intra-African; the only non-stop flights out of these three nations to Europe are operated by Air France and Brussels Airlines, heading for Paris, France and Brussels, Belgium, respectively.[38] Both airlines are members of an airline alliance that includes a U.S. carrier; members of an alliance often coordinate their services and have codeshare agreements.[39] For example, Thomas Eric Duncan, the first EVD patient diagnosed in the United States, reportedly flew on one ticket on a Brussels Airlines flight from Monrovia, Liberia to Belgium; a United Airlines flight from Belgium to Washington Dulles International Airport; and a United Airlines flight from Dulles to Dallas/Fort Worth.[40]

Travelers may not necessarily travel from the affected region to the United States on a single airline ticket. A passenger originating in one of the affected countries might travel to Europe on one ticket and book an entirely separate ticket, not necessarily on a code-sharing partner, to cross the Atlantic. In this case, the carrier flying the trans-Atlantic leg might not be aware that the travel originated in West Africa. It is also possible that a traveler could attempt to connect to the United States through airports in other African countries; however, many air and ground transportation links between the Ebola-affected countries and nearby countries have been suspended.[41]

On average, about 150 passengers travel from the three affected countries to the United States daily.[42] Among those, prior to October 21, 2014, 94% arrived at five major hub airports: John F. Kennedy International Airport (JFK); Newark Liberty International Airport (EWR); Washington Dulles International Airport (IAD); Hartsfield-Jackson Atlanta International Airport (ATL); and Chicago O'Hare International Airport (ORD).[43] On October 21, 2014, the Department of Homeland Security (DHS) announced that, effective October 22, 2014, all passengers arriving in the United States whose travel originates in Guinea, Liberia, or Sierra Leone are required to fly into one of the aforementioned five airports, which have enhanced screening procedures in place.[44] In addition, CDC and DHS announced that, effective November 17, 2014, entry screening would begin for travelers arriving from Mali, due to the evolving nature of outbreaks there. DHS states it will work with airlines to ensure that all passengers whose travel originates in Mali will enter the United States at one of the five airports discussed above.[45] DHS provides information about the number of arriving passengers screened, and the subset of them needing further assessment, on a public website.[46] For more information on screening procedures, see the subsequent section of this report, "How does entry screening in the United States work?"

### *Can the Federal Government Restrict the Use of U.S. Airspace?*[47]

The notion that each nation has complete and exclusive sovereignty over the airspace above its territory has been incorporated into international agreements dating back to the initial rise of international aviation.[48] Congress enshrined this principle in federal law in 1958, by declaring that "The United

States Government has exclusive sovereignty of airspace of the United States."[49] Congress delegated the authority to regulate U.S. airspace to the Administrator of the Federal Aviation Administration (FAA).[50] The FAA has the authority to restrict the use of U.S. airspace and prevent the entry of aircraft into U.S. airspace.[51] Additionally, the FAA has the authority to prevent U.S. carriers and operators from flying to or within the airspace of other countries.[52] In regulating the use of airspace for the benefit of the public interest, the FAA must consider several factors as being in the public interest, including "assigning, maintaining, and enhancing safety and security as the highest priorities in air commerce" and "regulating air commerce in a way that best promotes safety and fulfills national defense requirements."[53]

During the current Ebola outbreak, the FAA has acknowledged its authority to restrict the use of U.S. airspace, but has cautioned that decisions made on a public health basis would involve other federal agencies.[54] The FAA has stated:

> While the FAA has the authority to direct flight operations in United States airspace, any decision to restrict flights between the United States and other countries due to public health and disease concerns would be an interagency decision that would engage the Departments of Health and Human Services/CDC, State, Homeland Security, and Transportation.[55]

CRS has been unable to identify any instances in which the FAA has restricted the use of U.S. airspace by incoming or outgoing flights purely on the basis of a public health concern.

### *Can the Federal Government Prevent a Specific Person with a Communicable Disease from Boarding a U.S.-Bound Airplane?*[56]

DHS and CDC maintain a public health "Do Not Board" (DNB) list, which contains the names of people who are likely to be contagious with a communicable disease, may not adhere to public health recommendations, and are likely to board an aircraft.[57] Airlines are not permitted to issue a boarding pass to people on the DNB list for flights departing from or arriving into the United States. People placed on the DNB list are also "assigned a public health lookout record," which will alert CBP officers in the event the person attempts to enter the country through a port of entry.[58]

### *What if the Flight Crew Sees Someone Sick on Board an Aircraft?*[59]

Federal law requires a ship master or aircraft commander to immediately report a death on board or any ill person among the passengers and crew to a quarantine station nearest the port or airport of arrival.[60] For aircraft, such required reports are to be made to air traffic control and "[o]nce the FAA receives [the] report, it promptly communicates it to the CDC Emergency Operations Center."[61] Therefore, if the flight crew of a commercial aircraft arriving in the U.S. becomes aware of an ill person on board, which could include a person with Ebola symptoms, federal law requires the flight's commander to notify the nearest quarantine station. The CDC now also requests that airline crews ask sick travelers if they were in Guinea, Liberia, or Sierra Leone in the prior 21 days, and to report this information to CDC immediately.[62] The CDC maintains quarantine stations at 20 ports of entry and land-border crossings, including at international airports in the following areas: Atlanta, Chicago, Detroit, Honolulu, Houston, Los Angeles, Miami, Minneapolis-St. Paul, New York City (JFK), Philadelphia, San Francisco, San Juan, Seattle, and Washington, DC (IAD).[63]

### *What Other Steps Are Airlines and Airports Taking to Prevent the Spread of Ebola?*[64]

An airline operating any U.S.-bound flight may deny boarding to a customer that has a communicable disease or infection and poses a "direct threat," in accordance with Department of Transportation regulations.[65]

There are no enforceable federal regulations or standards regarding the cleaning or disinfecting of aircraft cabins or airport facilities. However, CDC issues non-binding guidance,[66] as does the Occupational Safety and Health Administration (OHSA).[67] In general, airlines follow certain CDC and OSHA guidelines, in addition to having internal protocols for aircraft cleaning. Additionally, WHO provides voluntary guidelines for hygiene and sanitation of airliners and airports.[68] Reportedly, U.S. carriers have tightened their aircraft cleaning regimens for aircraft arriving into the United States from West Africa to conform to WHO guidelines.[69] At some airports, infectious disease training has been offered to cleaning personnel, but concerns remain over training standards and the availability of appropriate cleaning supplies and suitable personal protective equipment for airport and aircraft cleaning crews.[70]

Major airports maintain biologic and pandemic incident response plans. The National Incident Management System[71] and the National Strategy for Pandemic Influenza[72] served as models for most of these airport plans.

However, some research has indicated that these protocols and guidelines are not always effectively followed and often have not been independently validated or tested.[73]

## Identification and Screening of Passengers Arriving from Ebola-Affected Countries

### *How Does Entry Screening in the United States Work?*[74]

Customs and Border Protection (CBP) conducts pre-travel electronic screening of all persons (including U.S. citizens) seeking to travel to the United States by air.[75] Starting 72 hours before the flight and prior to securing aircraft doors before departure, CBP receives data from commercial airlines (e.g., the Passenger Name Record [PNR] systems data[76] and the passenger and crew manifests[77]) and uses it to identify passengers who may be a risk to the United States (e.g., terrorists, criminals, and currently, those who have traveled from Guinea, Liberia, Sierra Leone, or Mali).[78]

As noted in the earlier section "How might people travel from affected countries to the United States?", persons whose travel originates in Guinea, Liberia, Sierra Leone, or Mali must enter the United States through one of five airports that have established new screening procedures for these passengers: John F. Kennedy International; Newark Liberty International; Washington Dulles; Atlanta Hartsfield-Jackson International, and Chicago O'Hare. When a passenger (including a U.S. citizen) whose travel originated in one of the four countries arrives, the passenger is escorted to a separate area for additional screening, fills out an extensive questionnaire, and has his or her temperature taken. If there are any concerns, CBP refers the person to CDC personnel at the airport who decide whether the person should be quarantined or allowed to continue to the final destination.[79] Travelers without fever or symptoms consistent with EVD are required to be monitored daily by the state and local health authorities for 21 days from the date of their departure from West Africa.[80] This is discussed more in the section "Who enforces monitoring and movement restrictions for those exposed to EVD?" Although entry screening has identified a number of persons who are ill upon arrival, no cases of EVD have been identified.[81]

### *What Are Other Countries Doing to Prevent the Introduction of Ebola via Air Travel?*[82]

Numerous countries around the world, including in Africa, have prohibited or restricted the issuance of visas to, or otherwise barred the entry of travelers from, the affected countries, or are screening travelers upon entry. A private medical travel and security company, International SOS, maintains a website that provides information on countries imposing travel restrictions on travelers originating from the affected countries.[83]

No European Union (EU) member states have barred travel from Ebola-affected countries, but some EU countries are screening travelers arriving from these countries.[84] There is no EU-wide policy regarding the entry of nationals from EVD-affected countries into the EU. Travel to EU countries is controlled by the authorities of each member state based on its own laws and regulations, which in most cases comply with common EU agreements and regulations. Most EU countries rely on the advice of EU health authorities, principally the European Centre for Disease Prevention and Control (ECDC). The ECDC maintains that "the added value of entry screening, if exit screening is being conducted effectively, is likely to be very small, and the resource implications considerable."[85] It also states, however, that "complementing exit screening with entry screening may, however, be considered: When there are doubts about the efficiency of exit screening [; and] to detect the few who may develop fever between the time of departure and the time of arrival."[86]

## Domestic Quarantine and Isolation: Legal Authority and Policies

### *What Is Quarantine? What Is Isolation?*[87]

Quarantine and isolation are different but related procedures to prevent the spread of infection. *Quarantine* is used to separate and restrict the movement of well persons who may have been exposed to a communicable disease, in case they become contagious. *Isolation* is used to separate ill persons who have a communicable disease from others, including their caregivers, to some extent. Isolation is often carried out in a healthcare setting.

### *What Legal Authority Allows the Federal Government to Quarantine or Isolate a Person?*[88]

The primary authority for communicable disease quarantine and isolation rests with states as an exercise of their traditional police powers.[89] However, the federal government has authority to order isolation and/or quarantine measures in certain situations. The Secretary of Health and Human Services is authorized to take measures "to prevent the introduction, transmission, or spread of communicable diseases from foreign countries into the States or possessions, or from one State or possession into any other State or possession."[90] The Secretary has delegated part of this responsibility to CDC, which is authorized to detain, isolate, or quarantine individuals suspected of carrying certain communicable diseases arriving from a foreign country, traveling from state-to-state, or believed to be a likely source of infection for individuals traveling to another state. However, such measures are limited to addressing communicable diseases published in an executive order issued by the President.[91] Executive Order 13295[92] lists the communicable diseases for which this quarantine authority may be exercised.[93] (The list includes Ebola.) Both interstate and foreign quarantine measures are now carried out by CDC's Division of Global Migration and Quarantine.[94]

There are currently 20 CDC Quarantine Stations located at ports of entry into the United States.[95] Because there are not CDC officials at every port of entry, various agencies in the Department of Homeland Security (DHS) are authorized to assist the CDC in "the enforcement of quarantine rules and regulations."[96] If an individual is suspected of carrying a communicable disease specified by the President, CDC may issue an isolation or quarantine order, a violation of which is a criminal misdemeanor.[97]

### *What Does the Federal Government Recommend for Persons Exposed to EVD?*[98]

CDC has revised its guidance for the management of persons who may have been exposed to EVD in order to prevent spread of the disease, should an exposed person become ill and contagious.[99] These guidelines address travelers from Ebola-affected countries in Africa as well as contacts potentially exposed to EVD within the United States.

The guidance distinguishes between *persons with symptoms* of illness and those without (i.e., *persons who are asymptomatic*). Persons with possible EVD exposure who are ill may be contagious to others and should be isolated and evaluated by medical and public health personnel immediately, according to protocols that prevent transmission of the disease to others.

Persons who have potentially been *exposed to Ebola virus* but have no symptoms of illness are not contagious to others. The incubation period for EVD, the time between exposure and the development of symptoms (i.e., the onset of illness), ranges from 2 to 21 days; in most cases it falls between 9 to

11 days.[100] After 21 days a person who was potentially exposed to Ebola virus but has not become ill is very unlikely to do so.

The CDC guidance defines several *levels of risk of exposure* among asymptomatic persons. These levels, and some examples of persons at each level, are

- *High risk*: direct contact with body fluids, or the dead body, of an infected person (including a needlestick injury or other known breach of personal protective equipment, PPE); living with and caring for an infected person.
- *Some risk*: care of an infected person in a country with widespread transmission (i.e., Guinea, Liberia, or Sierra Leone) or in Mali while using PPE properly.
- *Low risk:* care of an infected person in a country without widespread transmission while using PPE properly; being in a country with widespread transmission or in Mali within the prior 21 days.
- *No risk:* contact with another asymptomatic person who cares for someone with EVD infection, or who later develops EVD; persons traveling from a country (other than Mali) that has had Ebola cases but not widespread transmission.[101]

For those at risk of exposure, the CDC guidance stresses frequent (at least once daily) *monitoring for symptoms* such as fever, headache, vomiting, or diarrhea, among others. The premise is that if an exposed person is isolated promptly upon the onset of symptoms, there will have been no transmission of the virus to others. The exposure level determines whether monitoring is carried out directly by a public health worker, verified by phone or other electronic communication with a health worker, or is simply documented by the potentially exposed person. In any case, persons who develop symptoms while under monitoring are to report to public health officials immediately and facilitate prompt isolation measures.

Along with careful monitoring, *movement restrictions* such as home quarantine may be recommended as secondary control measures. The guidance does not advise strict quarantine in a specified location for most exposure risk levels, although at higher exposure levels it recommends "controlled movement," such as avoiding mass transit and mass gatherings.[102] The guidance suggests that movement restrictions can be crafted by public health officials on a case by case basis for many potentially exposed persons.

### *How Does the Current Guidance Differ from the Prior Version?*[103]

The current (November 16) guidance supersedes guidance published on August 22,[104] and recommends that all healthcare workers who care for EVD patients should be considered at low or some risk of EVD exposure, even if they have used PPE with no known breach. In addition, persons having traveled from severely affected countries (i.e., Guinea, Liberia, or Sierra Leone) or to Mali should be considered at low risk even if they have no known close contact with an Ebola patient. Finally, U.S. state and local public health officials are urged to conduct active monitoring of at-risk persons during their 21-day monitoring period.[105]

### *Who Enforces Monitoring and Movement Restrictions for Those Exposed to EVD?*[106]

In general, state and local public health officials are responsible for setting the terms of monitoring and movement restrictions for exposed persons, as an exercise of their police powers. (See the earlier section, "What legal authority allows the federal government to quarantine or isolate a person?".)

State and local health officials are directly involved in tracing, identifying, and managing contacts when Ebola transmission may have occurred in the United States. Entrants (travelers) identified by CDC or CBP officials as having possible exposure are required to provide information about their final U.S. destination, and contact information. CDC or CBP officials then provide this information to public health officials at the final destination, who commence the daily monitoring and any additional protocols recommended for these persons.[107]

If a traveler with the potential for EVD exposure is found to be ill upon arrival in the United States, CDC or CBP officials may, pursuant to CDC's quarantine authority, require the person to be immediately isolated and transported to a nearby hospital for further evaluation.

In addition, if federal or state/local officials determine that an asymptomatic but potentially exposed individual should not travel by air once at the final U.S. destination, CDC and CBP may place the individual on the Do Not Board list for the duration of the person's quarantine period, as discussed in the previous section of this report, "Can the federal government prevent a specific person with a communicable disease from boarding a U.S.-bound airplane?".

### *How Do States Enforce Monitoring Requirements and Movement Restrictions?*[108]

All states have the authority and the legal means to require monitoring and movement restriction of individuals in order to ensure public health and safety. State laws and procedures vary considerably in their particulars, however.[109]

Following the 2001 terrorist attacks, CDC funding was provided to aid states in their public health preparedness efforts,[110] which included updating their quarantine laws and otherwise improving their legal preparedness for infectious disease threats. Specifically, CDC funded development of a model state emergency health powers act for states to adopt, in whole or part.[111] In 2011, CDC published *Public Health Preparedness Capabilities: National Standards for State and Local Planning* (PHEP Capabilities) to help state and local planners identify and address gaps in their readiness for public health threats.[112] The document presents "priority elements" that should be addressed in a state's or locality's written public health emergency plan, including the following regarding isolation and quarantine capability:

> ...documentation of the applicable jurisdictional, legal, and regulatory authorities and policies for recommending and implementing non-pharmaceutical interventions in both routine and incident-specific situations. This includes but is not limited to authorities for restricting the following elements: [Individuals; Groups; Facilities; Animals (e.g., animals with infectious diseases and animals with exposure to environmental, chemical, radiological hazards); Consumer food products; Public works/utilities (e.g., water supply); and Travel through ports of entry].[113]

### *How Has the Public Reacted to U.S. Quarantine Policies?*[114]

A CBS News poll conducted in late October, 2014, found that 80% of Americans think that asymptomatic U.S. citizens and legal residents returning from West Africa should be quarantined upon their arrival in the United States until it is certain they don't have Ebola infection.[115]

Aid groups and others have cautioned that forced quarantine could dissuade healthcare workers from volunteering for Ebola response missions in West Africa.[116] CDC guidance does not generally recommend quarantine for potentially Ebola-exposed persons who do not have symptoms. (See the earlier section "What does the federal government recommend for persons exposed to EVD?".) However, the Department of Defense has imposed a 21-day quarantine on military members deployed to Ebola-affected countries in West Africa, upon their return.[117]

Quarantine can be cumbersome, intrusive, and fraught with unintended consequences, but, when applied skillfully, it is a time-tested approach to stopping the spread of communicable diseases.[118] Decisions to use or forgo quarantine are likely to continue to stir debate in American communities, regardless of the science behind them or the passage of time, because these decisions reveal the nation's diverse views about the balance of individual and collective wellbeing.[119]

## End Notes

[1] Contributed by Michael John Garcia, Legislative Attorney, 7-3873, mgarcia@crs.loc.gov, and Alison Siskin, Specialist in Immigration Policy, 7-0260, asiskin@crs.loc.gov.

[2] Authorities to except or to waive visa requirements are specified in law, such as the broad parole authority of the Secretary of Homeland Security under §212(d)(5) of the Immigration and Nationality Act (INA) and the specific authority of the Visa Waiver Program in INA §217. See CRS Report R41104, Immigration Visa Issuances and Grounds for Exclusion: Policy and Trends, by Ruth Ellen Wasem.

[3] See, e.g., Landon v. Plasencia, 459 U.S. 21, 32 (1982) ("an alien seeking admission to the United States requests a privilege and has no constitutional rights regarding his application, for the power to admit or exclude aliens is a sovereign prerogative.... ").

[4] Having a valid visa does not guarantee admittance to the United States. At ports of entry, foreign nationals are screened by Customs and Border Protection (CBP) to make sure that they are not inadmissible according to the specified grounds in the INA, including health-related grounds.

[5] Immigration and Nationality Act (INA) §212(a)(1), 8 U.S.C. §1182(a)(1).

[6] The Secretary of Health and Human Services is responsible for defining illnesses constituting a "communicable disease of public health significance." Current regulations define the term to include, among other things, those diseases listed in a Presidential Executive Order or subject to specified requirements under the rules of the World Health Organization. 42 C.F.R. §34.2. Due to practical concerns, a foreign national arriving at a U.S. port of entry who is believed to have the Ebola virus would be placed in isolation and given medical treatment, rather than immediately being placed in removal proceedings or given the option of promptly leaving the United States.

[7] Foreign nationals with lawful permanent resident (LPR) status are authorized to permanently live in the United States. They are also eligible to work in the United States.

[8] See INA §101(a)(13)(C), 8 U.S.C. §1101(a)(13)(C) (exempting most lawful permanent residents who are returning to the United States after brief trips abroad from being viewed as seeking admission into the country).

[9] INA §212(f), 8 U.S.C. §1182(f) (broadly permitting the President to "suspend the entry of all aliens or any class of aliens as immigrants or nonimmigrants, or impose on the entry of aliens any restrictions he may deem to be appropriate").

[10] A list of presidential proclamations pursuant to INA §212(f) which are currently in effect can be viewed at http://travel.state.gov/content/visas/english/fees/presidential-proclamations.html. For further discussion regarding the potential use of INA §212(f) to restrict the travel of foreign nationals from Ebola-stricken countries, see CRS Legal Sidebar WSLG1094, Can the President Bar Foreign Travelers from Ebola-Stricken Countries from Entering the United States? by Michael John Garcia.

[11] For a list of the current closed consulates and embassies, see U.S. Department of State, Countries with Limited or No U.S. Visa Services, http://travel.state.gov/content/visas/english/general/countries-with-limited-or-no-u-s—visaservices.html.

[12] In August 2009, the U.S. Embassy in Honduras temporarily suspended issuing nonimmigrant, non-emergency visas to put pressure on the government there to reinstate the deposed president, Manuel Zelaya. Department of State, "Temporary Suspension of Non-Immigrant Visa Services in Honduras," press release, August 25, 2009, http://www.state.gov/r/pa/prs/ps/2009/aug/128349.htm.

[13] In the summer of 2014, for example, the U.S. Embassy in Tel Aviv, Israel, reduced its staff due to security concerns, and as a result canceled the processing of nonimmigrant visas except in emergency situations. The embassy also suspended routine services to U.S. citizens.

[14] For example, visa services at the U.S. Consulate in Calgary were limited for the month of November 2014 due to building renovations. See United States Consulate General in Calgary, Announcement, Oct. 16, 2014, available at http://calgary.usconsulate.gov/news-events/consulate-news-and-events/2014/limited-consular-services-in-november2014.html.

[15] See footnote 11 (listing closed embassies and consular offices and providing instructions for where affected foreign nationals may apply for a visa).

[16] B-visas (short-term visas for business or tourism), for instance, are valid for a period of 36 months for nationals of Sierra Leone and Guinea and for a year for nationals of Liberia.

[17] See for example WHO, "Ebola Travel Advice: WHO Does Not Recommend General Bans on Travel or Trade," http://www.who.int/csr/disease/ebola/travel-advice/en/.

[18] Dr. Isabelle Nuttall, Director, Global Capacities, Alert and Response, WHO, "Ebola Travel: Vigilance, Not Bans," Commentary, November 5, 2014, http://www.who.int/mediacentre/commentaries/ebola-travel/en/.

[19] Different types of visas are issued for different purposes. Immigrant visas are issued to those intending to live permanently in the United States, and nonimmigrant visas to those coming to the United States for a specific purpose and specified period of time. The 72 categories of nonimmigrant visas include B-visas for short-term visitors for business or tourism, H-visas for temporary workers, F-visas for students, and L-visas for intercompany transfers. CRS Report R41104, Immigration Visa Issuances and Grounds for Exclusion: Policy and Trends, by Ruth Ellen Wasem.

[20] Weekly federal interagency Ebola update call for Congressional staff, October 16, 2014.

[21] Some federal courts have found that the right of an American citizen to return to the United States from abroad is a substantive due process right. See Fikre v. F.B.I., 3:13-CV-00899-BR, 2014 WL 2335343 (D. Or. May 29, 2014); Tarhuni v. Holder, 3:13-CV-00001-BR, 2014 WL 1269655 (D. Or. Mar. 26, 2014); see also Nguyen v. Immigration and Naturalization Serv., 533 U.S. 53, 67 (2001) (discussing privileges of U.S. citizenship, including "the absolute right to enter [the] borders" of the United States).

[22] Contributed by Tiaji Salaam-Blyther, Specialist in Global Health, 7-7677, tsalaam@crs.loc.gov, and Nicolas Cook, Specialist in African Affairs, 7-0429, ncook@crs.loc.gov.

[23] WHO, "Ebola Virus Disease Exit Screening at Airports, Ports and Land Crossings: Interim Guidance," November 6, 2014, p. 4, referencing WHO guidance of August 2014, http://www.who.int/csr/resources/publications/ebola/exitscreening-guidance/en/. WHO provides EVD case definition guidelines for the purpose of making EVD detection assessments. See WHO, "Case Definition Recommendations for Ebola or Marburg Virus Diseases," August 9, 2014, http://www.who.int/csr/resources/publications/ebola/ebola-case-definition-contact-en.pdf.

[24] WHO, "Travel and Transport Risk Assessment: Interim Guidance for Public Health Authorities and the Transport Sector," September 2014, http://www.who.int/csr/resources/publications/ebola/travel-guidance/en/.

[25] Ibid.

[26] CDC, "Ebola Virus Disease (Ebola) Pre-Departure/Exit Screening at Points of Departure in Affected Countries," Version 9, August 30, 2014, http://wwwnc.cdc.gov/travel/page/ebola-outbreak-communication-resources. Appendix 4 of the guide provides a sample exit screening questionnaire.

[27] Ibid, p. 5.

[28] USAID, "West Africa Ebola Outbreak," Fact Sheet #3, October 14, 2014, http://www.usaid.gov/ebola/fy15/fs03.

[29] UN Mission for Ebola Emergency Response (UNMEER) External Situation Report, October 17, 2014, http://www.un.org/ebolaresponse/resources.shtml.

[30] CRS Report R43750, Ebola: Basics About the Disease, by Sarah A. Lister.

[31] Ibid.

[32] Isaac I. Bogoch, et al., "Assessment of the Potential for International Dissemination of Ebola Virus via Commercial Air Travel During the 2014 West African Outbreak," The Lancet, October 21, 2014, http://ebola.thelancet.com/.

[33] WHO, "Travel and Transport Risk Assessment: Interim Guidance for Public Health Authorities and the Transport Sector," September 2014, p. 6, http://who.int/csr/resources/publications/ebola/travel-guidance/en/. This WHO guide provides for purposes of public education a "Template message for travelers" that provides basic information about the disease, modes of EVD infection and its prevention, and related information.

[34] WHO, "Statement from the Travel and Transport Task Force on Ebola Virus Disease Outbreak in West Africa," November 7, 2014, http://who.int/mediacentre/news/ statements/2014/ebola-travel/en/.

[35] Contributed by Rachel Tang, Analyst in Transportation and Industry, 7-7875, rtang@crs.loc.gov.

[36] Data provided by and discussion with Airlines for America, an industry association representing major U.S. air carriers. This has been confirmed by the Department of Transportation and the Department of Homeland Security.

[37] Ibid.

[38] Ibid.

[39] Brussels Airlines is a member of the Star Alliance network, along with U.S. carrier United Airlines. Star Alliance, "Travel the World with the Star Alliance Network," http://www.staralliance.com/en/about/member_airlines/. Air France is a member of the SkyTeam network, along with U.S. carrier Delta Airlines. SkyTeam, "SkyTeam Members," https://www.skyteam.com/en/About-us/Our-members/.

[40] Larry Buchanan et al., "Retracing the Steps of the Dallas Ebola Patient," N.Y. Times, October 8, 2014.

[41] Voice of America News, "Airlines Cut West Africa Flights, Delay Ebola Aid," September 12, 2014, http://www.voanews.com/content/airlines-cuts-in-flights-to-west-africa-delay-ebola-aid/2448006.html; Achilleas Galatsidas and Mark Anderson, "West Africa in Quarantine: Ebola, Closed Borders and Travel Bans," The Guardian, August 22, 2014, http://www.theguardian.com/global-development/ng-interactive/2014/aug/22/ebola-west-africaclosed-borders-travel-bans; see also International SOS, "Travel restrictions, flight operations, and screening," November 3, 2014, https://www.internationalsos.com/ebola/index.cfm?content_id=435&.

[42] Andrew Grossman, Carol E. Lee, and Jack Nicas, "U.S. to Check Temperatures of West Africa Passengers at Five Airports," Wall Street Journal, October 8, 2014.

[43] The White House Blog, "Five U.S. Airports Are Enacting New Screening Measures to Protect Against Ebola," October 8, 2014, http://www.whitehouse.gov/blog/2014/10/08/five-us-airports-are-enacting-new-screening-measuresprotect-against-ebola.

[44] DHS, "Statement by Secretary Johnson on Travel Restrictions and Protective Measures to Prevent the Spread of Ebola to the United States," press release, October 21, 2014, http://www.dhs.gov/news-releases/press-releases.

[45] CDC and DHS, "Enhanced Airport Entry Screening to Begin for Travelers to the United States from Mali," press release, November 16, 2014, http://www.cdc.gov/media/ archives.htm.

[46] DHS, "DHS's Coordinated Response to Ebola," http://www.dhs.gov/ebola-response.

[47] Contributed by Alissa M. Dolan, Legislative Attorney, 7-8433, adolan@crs.loc.gov.

[48] See, e.g., Convention for the Regulation of Aerial Navigation (Paris Convention), Oct. 13, 1919, Art. 1; Convention on International Civil Aviation (Chicago Convention), Dec. 7, 1944, Art. 1.

[49] 49 U.S.C. §40103(a).

[50] 49 U.S.C. §40103(b).

[51] See 49 U.S.C. §§40103(b), 44701. FAA issues Notice to Airmen (NOTAM) to announce temporary flight restrictions in U.S. airspace according to FAA regulation. See 14 C.F.R. §§91.137-138, 91.141, 91.143-145.

[52] See 49 U.S.C. §§40101(d)(1), 44701(a)(5). For an example of such a restriction, see "Prohibition Against Certain Flights Within the Territory and Airspace of Somalia," 72 Fed. Reg. 16710 (April 5, 2007).

[53] 49 U.S.C. §40101(d)(1).

[54] Federal Aviation Administration (FAA), "FAA Statement on Ebola," press release, Oct. 3, 2014, http://www.faa.gov/ news/press_releases/.

[55] Id.

[56] Contributed by Jared P. Cole, Legislative Attorney, 7-6350, jpcole@crs.loc.gov.

[57] See CDC, "Federal Air Travel Restrictions for Public Health Purposes—United States, June 2007-May 2008," MMWR, September 19, 2008, http://www.cdc.gov/mmwr/preview/mmwrhtml/mm5737a1.htm.

[58] Id.

[59] Contributed by Alissa M. Dolan, Legislative Attorney, 7-8433, adolan@crs.loc.gov.

[60] 42 C.F.R. §71.21. For ships, the reporting requirement covers a death or illness that occurs within 15 days prior to the date of expected arrival or since departure from a U.S. port, whichever time period is shorter.

[61] Federal Aviation Administration (FAA), "FAA Statement on Ebola," press release, October 3, 2014, http://www.faa.gov/news/press_releases/.

[62] CDC, "Guidance for Airlines on Reporting Onboard Deaths or Illnesses to CDC," October 15, 2014, http://www.cdc.gov/quarantine/air/reporting-deaths-illness/guidance-reporting-onboard-deaths-illnesses.html.

[63] CDC, "Quarantine Station Contact List, Map, and Fact Sheets," http://www.cdc.gov/quarantine/ quarantinestationcontactlistfull.html.

[64] Contributed by Bart Elias, Specialist in Aviation Policy, 7-7771, belias@crs.loc.gov.

[65] See 14 C.F.R. §382.21. A "direct threat" means a "significant risk to the health or safety of others that cannot be eliminated by a modification of policies, practices, or procedures, or by the provision of auxiliary aids or services." 14 C.F.R. §382.3.

[66] CDC, "Ebola Guidance for Airlines: Interim Guidance about Ebola Infection for Airline Crews, Cleaning Personnel, and Cargo Personnel," http://wwwnc.cdc.gov/travel/page/travel-industry-information-center.

[67] OSHA, "Ebola: Control and Prevention," https://www.osha.gov/SLTC/ ebola/control_prevention.html.

[68] WHO, "Guide to Hygiene and Sanitation in Aviation," Third ed. 2009, http://www.who.int/water_sanitation_health/hygiene/ships/guide_hygiene_sanitation_aviation_3_edition.pdf.

[69] Scott McCartney, "The Trouble with Keeping Commercial Flights Clean," Wall Street Journal, September 17, 2014.

[70] Bart Jansen, "Airport Workers Ill-Equipped to Cope with Sick Fliers," USA Today, October 8, 2014, http://www.usatoday.com/story/news/nation/2014/10/08/airport-cleaners-seiu-jfk-laguardia/16909177/.

[72] See Flu.gov, "Planning and Preparedness," http://www.flu.gov/planning-preparedness/federal/index.html.

[73] Duane Habeck, "Communications and Information Management Issues for Air Travel Disease Mitigation," Federal Roles in Air Travel Disease Mitigation, Transportation Research Board 2014 Annual Meeting.

[74] Contributed by Alison Siskin, Specialist in Immigration Policy, 7-0260, asiskin@crs.loc.gov.

[75] For a fuller discussion of CBP's air passenger screening procedures, see CRS Report R43356, Border Security: Immigration Inspections at Ports of Entry, by Lisa Seghetti.

[76] 19 C.F.R. §122.49d. The data include passport and travel itinerary information.

[77] 19 C.F.R. §§122.49a, 122.49b.

[78] CBP, "Frequently Asked Questions, U.S. Customs and Border Protection, Receipt of Passenger Name Record (PNR) Data," June 21, 2013, http://www.cbp.gov/sites/ default/files/documents/pnr_faq_3.pdf.

[79] This referral is referred to as "tertiary" (i.e., the third) inspection.

[80] Post-arrival monitoring began in the six states (Georgia, Maryland, New Jersey, New York, Pennsylvania, and Virginia) where approximately 70% of travelers are headed. CDC, "CDC Announces Active Post-Arrival Monitoring for Travelers from Impacted Countries," press release, October 22, 2014, http://www.cdc.gov/media/archives.htm.

[81] DHS, "DHS's Coordinated Response to Ebola," http://www.dhs.gov/ebola-response.

[82] Contributed by Tiaji Salaam-Blyther, Specialist in Global Health, 7-7677, tsalaam@crs.loc.gov, and Nicolas Cook, Specialist in African Affairs, 7-0429, ncook @crs.loc.gov.

[83] International SOS, "Travel Restrictions, Flight Operations and Screening," among other Ebola-related resources at https://www.internationalsos.com/ebola/. Information is updated regularly but does not consistently reflect all current travel restrictions.

[84] Adrian Croft and Francesco Guarascio, "EU Disagrees on Need for Ebola Screening at Europe's Airports," Reuters, October 16, 2014; and AFP, "Brussels Becomes Latest EU Airport to Screen for Ebola," October 20, 2014.

[85] European Centre for Disease Prevention and Control (ECDC), "Infection Prevention and Control Measures for Ebola Virus Disease Entry and Exit Screening Measures, Technical Report," October 12, 2014, http://www.ecdc.europa.eu/ en/publications/technical_reports/ Pages/index.aspx.

[86] Ibid. The ECDC also reported that, as of mid-October 2014, no information was "available regarding the quality and performance of the exit screening implemented in the affected countries," and has identified several aspects of both exit and entry screening that indicate that screening may result in a failure to detect EVD. See ECDC, Outbreak of Ebola Virus Disease in West Africa, Rapid Risk Assessment, Seventh update, October 17, 2014.

[87] Contributed by Sarah A. Lister, Specialist in Public Health and Epidemiology, 7-7320, slister@crs.loc.gov.

[88] Contributed by Jared P. Cole, Legislative Attorney, 7-6350, jpcole@crs.loc.gov.

[89] See Compagnie Francaise de Navigation a Vapeur v. Louisiana State Board of Health, 186 U.S. 380 (1902). "Police power" refers to the power of a state to establish and enforce laws protecting the welfare, safety, and health of the public. See Patterson v. State of Kentucky, 97 U.S. 501, 504 (1878); Mugler v. Kansas, 123 U.S. 623 (1887).

[90] 42 U.S.C. §264.

[91] 42 U.S.C. §264(b).

[92] See Exec. Order No. 13674, 79 Fed. Reg. 45671 (August 6, 2014); Exec. Order No. 13375, 70 Fed. Reg. 17299 (April 1, 2005).

[93] Exec. Order No. 13295, 68 Fed. Reg. 17255 (April 4, 2003). The diseases currently listed are cholera, diphtheria, infectious tuberculosis, plague, smallpox, yellow fever, viral hemorrhagic fevers (including Ebola), severe acute respiratory syndrome (SARS), and influenza viruses which have the potential to cause a pandemic.

[94] Whether an isolation or quarantine order originates with the federal or state government, such orders will presumably be subject to habeas corpus challenges, and must also comport with the Due Process Clause of the Constitution. See CRS Report RL33201, Federal and State Quarantine and Isolation Authority, by Jared P. Cole.

[95] See Centers for Disease Control and Prevention (CDC), U.S. Quarantine Stations, http://www. cdc.gov/quarantine/ quarantine-stations-us.html.

[96] 42 U.S.C. §268.

[97] 42 U.S.C. §271.

[98] Contributed by Sarah A. Lister, Specialist in Public Health and Epidemiology, 7-7320, slister@crs.loc.gov.

[99] CDC, "Interim U.S. Guidance for Monitoring and Movement of Persons with Potential Ebola Virus Exposure," October 28, 2014 (updated November 16, 2014), http://www.cdc.gov/ vhf/ebola/exposure/monitoring-and-movementof-persons-with-exposure.html.

[100] CDC, "Ebola Virus Disease Information for Clinicians in U.S. Healthcare Settings," November 9, 2014, http://www.cdc.gov/vhf/ebola/hcp/clinician-information-us-healthcare-settings.html.

[101] CDC, "Questions and Answers about CDC's Ebola Monitoring and Movement Guidance," November 8, 2014, http://www.cdc.gov/vhf/ebola/exposure/qas-monitoring-and-movement-guidance.html.

[102] CDC, "Interim U.S. Guidance for Monitoring and Movement of Persons with Potential Ebola Virus Exposure," October 28, 2014 (updated November 16, 2014), http://www.cdc.gov/vhf/ebola/exposure/monitoring-and-movementof-persons-with-exposure.html.

[103] Contributed by Sarah A. Lister, Specialist in Public Health and Epidemiology, 7-7320, slister@crs.loc.gov.

[104] CDC, "Interim Guidance for Monitoring and Movement of Persons with Ebola Virus Disease Exposure," updated August 22, 2014.

[105] CDC, "Questions and Answers about CDC's Ebola Monitoring and Movement Guidance," November 8, 2014, http://www.cdc.gov/vhf/ebola/exposure/qas-monitoring-and-movement-guidance.html.

[106] Contributed by Sarah A. Lister, Specialist in Public Health and Epidemiology, 7-7320, slister @crs.loc.gov.

[107] Department of Homeland Security, "DHS's Coordinated Response to Ebola," http://www.dhs.gov/ebola-response.

[108] Contributed by Sarah A. Lister, Specialist in Public Health and Epidemiology, 7-7320, slister@crs.loc.gov.

[109] See National Council of State Legislatures, "State Quarantine and Isolation Statutes," a database, updated October 29, 2014, http://www.ncsl.org/research/health/state-quarantine-and-isolation-statutes.aspx.

[110] CDC, "Funding and Guidance for State and Local Health Departments," http://www.cdc.gov/phpr/ coopagreement.htm.

[111] See "Model State Emergency Health Powers Act" in CRS Report RS21414, Mandatory Vaccinations: Precedent and Current Laws, by Jared P. Cole and Kathleen S. Swendiman.

[112] CDC, Public Health Preparedness Capabilities: National Standards for State and Local Planning, July 22, 2011, http://www.cdc.gov/phpr/capabilities/.

[113] Ibid, pp. 102-103. In contrast to drugs and vaccines, "non-pharmaceutical interventions" for communicable disease control refer to restrictions such isolation and quarantine, and other interventions such as cancellation of large events.

[114] Contributed by Sarah A. Lister, Specialist in Public Health and Epidemiology, 7-7320, slister@crs.loc.gov.

[115] Sarah Dutton, et al., "Do Americans Believe there Should Be a Quarantine to Deal with Ebola?" CBS News, October 29, 2014, http://www.cbsnews.com/feature/cbs-news-polls/.

[116] See for example Doctors Without Borders/Médecins Sans Frontières (MSF), "Ebola: Quarantine Can Undermine Efforts to Curb Epidemic," press release, October 27, 2014, http://www.doctorswithoutborders.org/news-stories/press/ press-releases.

[117] See for example Dion Nissenbaum, "Hagel Approves 21-Day Ebola Isolation Period for Military; Applies to All Servicemembers Returning from West Africa," The Wall Street Journal, October 30, 2014.

[118] See for example Jon Schuppe, "Dallas Ebola Family Joins Long History of Quarantines," NBC News, October 4, 2014.

[119] Kate Murphy, "The Ethics of Infection," The New York Times, November 8, 2014.

In: Ebola
Editor: MaryAnn Cole
ISBN: 978-1-63482-253-4


*Chapter 4*

# STATEMENT OF DR. THOMAS R. FRIEDEN, DIRECTOR, CENTERS FOR DISEASE CONTROL AND PREVENTION. HEARING ON "EXAMINING THE U.S. PUBLIC HEALTH RESPONSE TO THE EBOLA OUTBREAK"*

Good afternoon Chairman Murphy, Ranking Member DeGette, and members of the Subcommittee. Thank you for the opportunity to testify before you today and for your ongoing support for the Centers for Disease Control and Prevention's (CDC) work in protecting Americans. I am Dr. Tom Frieden, Director of the CDC. I appreciate the opportunity to be here today to discuss the epidemic of Ebola, as well as the work the CDC is doing to manage the consequences of this epidemic – both here in the United States and overseas – in the wake of the first diagnosed case here in the United States two weeks ago, which ultimately and tragically has become the first death from Ebola in the United States. Additionally, I will address the work CDC and public health officials in Texas are undertaking in response to the transmission of Ebola to two health care workers here in the United States, which occurred this week.

From the time the situation in West Africa escalated from an outbreak to an epidemic, we have anticipated that a traveler could arrive in the United States with the disease. We have been preparing for this possibility by working closely with our state and local partners and with clinicians and health care

* This is an edited, reformatted and augmented version of a statement presented October 16, 2014 before the House Energy and Commerce Committee, Subcommittee on Oversight and Investigations.

facilities so that any imported case could be quickly contained. This occurrence underscores the need to carefully follow the protocols that have been developed, to work closely across levels of government, and to continue our urgent effort to address the epidemic in West Africa, which remains the biggest risk to the United States.

As we learn from the recent importation case in Dallas and subsequent transmissions, and continue the public health response there, we remain confident that Ebola is not a significant public health threat to the United States. It is not transmitted easily, and it does not spread from people who are not ill, and cultural norms that contribute to the spread of the disease in Africa – such as burial customs and inadequate public-health measures – are not a factor in the United States. We know Ebola can be stopped with rapid diagnosis, appropriate triage, and meticulous infection-control practices in American hospitals. And the United States is leading the international effort to stop it at the source in Africa. CDC is committing significant resources both on the ground in West Africa and through our Emergency Operations Center here at home.

We have been constantly monitoring our response in the United States, and will continue to do so. CDC and U.S. Customs and Border Protection (CBP) in the Department of Homeland Security (DHS) have implemented new layers of entry screening at five U.S. airports that receive over 94 percent of travelers from the Ebola-affected nations of Guinea, Liberia, and Sierra Leone. On October 11, 2014, we began screening New York's JFK International Airport, since in the 12 months ending July 2014, JFK received nearly half of all travelers from those three West African nations. The enhanced entry screening has expanded this week at Washington-Dulles, Newark, Chicago-O'Hare, and Atlanta international airports.

This is a whole-of-Government response, with agencies across the United States Government committing human and financial resources. Across HHS, CDC is actively partnering with the Office of Global Affairs, the Office of the Assistant Secretary for Preparedness and Response, the National Institutes of Health, and the Food and Drug Administration to coordinate and respond to this epidemic.

Also, CDC has embedded technical staff as the leads for the health, medical, and public health aspects of the response in the USAID-led DART team in West Africa. Additionally, staff, logistical support, and resources from the Department of Defense (DoD) are already being deployed to rapidly scale up our efforts to include constructing Ebola Treatment Units (ETUs) and training health care workers. We are working closely with our international partners to scale up the response to the levels needed to stop this epidemic.

Ebola is a severe, often fatal, viral hemorrhagic fever. The first Ebola virus was detected in 1976 in what is now the Democratic Republic of Congo. Since then, outbreaks have appeared sporadically. The current epidemic in Guinea, Liberia, and Sierra Leone is the first time an outbreak has been recognized in West Africa, the first-ever Ebola epidemic, and the biggest and most complex Ebola challenge the world has ever faced. We have seen cases imported into Nigeria and Senegal from the initially-affected areas and we have also seen in Nigeria and Senegal that proven practices such as contact tracing, monitoring, and isolation practices can contribute to managing Ebola and preventing a small number of cases from growing into a larger outbreak.

Ebola has symptoms similar to many other illnesses, including fever, chills, weakness and body aches. Gastrointestinal symptoms such as vomiting and diarrhea are common and profound, with fluid losses on average of 5-7 liters in 24 hours over a five day period. These fluid losses can result in life-threatening electrolyte losses. In approximately half of cases there is hemorrhage -- serious internal and external bleeding. There are two things that are very important to understand about how Ebola spreads. First, the current evidence suggests human-to-human transmission of Ebola only happens from people who are symptomatic– not from people who have been exposed to, but are not ill with the disease. Second, everything we have seen in our decades of experience with Ebola indicates that Ebola is not spread by casual contact; Ebola is spread through direct contact with bodily fluids of someone who is sick with, or has died from Ebola, or through exposure to objects such as needles that have been contaminated. While the illness has an average 8-10 day incubation period (though it may be as short as two days and as long as 21 days), we recommend monitoring for fever and signs of symptoms for the full 21 days. Again, we do not believe people are contagious during that incubation period, when they have no symptoms. Evidence does not suggest Ebola is spread through the air.

The earliest recorded cases in the current epidemic were reported in March of this year. Following an initial response that seemed to slow the early outbreak for a time, cases flared again due to weak systems of health care and public health and because of challenges health workers faced in dealing with communities where critical disease-control measures were in conflict with regular practices. As of last week, the epidemic has reached 8,997 reported cases, including 4,493 documented deaths, though we believe these numbers may be substantially under-reported. The effort to control the epidemic in some places is complicated by fear of the disease and distrust of outsiders. Security is tenuous and unstable, especially in remote isolated rural areas. There have been instances where public health teams could not do their jobs because of security concerns, although community outreach has resulted in acceptance of services in specific areas.

Many of the health systems in the affected countries in West Africa were weak prior to the Ebola outbreak, and do not reach into rural areas effectively. Health care workers are often too few in number and not reliably present at facilities, and those facilities have limited capacity. Poor infection control in routine health care in these three countries, along with traditions such as public funerals and preparing bodies of the deceased for burial, make efforts to contain the illness more difficult. Furthermore, the porous land borders among countries and remoteness of many villages have greatly complicated control efforts. The epidemic has further weakened these fragile healthcare systems – even to the point of collapse – and as a result local populations have lost access to treatment for other major health issues, such as malaria, diarrheal disease, or assistance with child delivery. The secondary effects of this outbreak also transcend the medical realm, as the economies of the affected countries have taken major blows that could impact their growth and development for years to come. The region also faces greater international isolation, and the potential for political instability. These impacts are intensifying, and not only signal a growing humanitarian crisis, but also have direct impacts on our ability to respond to the Ebola epidemic itself.

Fortunately, we know what we must do. In order to stop an Ebola outbreak, we must find active cases, respond appropriately, and prevent future cases. The use of real-time diagnostics is extremely important to identify new cases. We must support the strengthening of health systems and assist in training healthcare providers. Once active cases have been identified, we must support quality patient care in treatment centers, prevent further transmission through proper infection control practices, and protect healthcare workers. Epidemiologists must identify contacts of infected patients and follow up with them every day for 21 days, initiating testing and isolation if symptoms emerge. And, we must intensify our use of health communication tools to disseminate messages about effective prevention and risk reduction. These messages include recommendations to report suspected cases, to avoid close contact with sick people or the deceased, and to promote safe burial practices. In Africa, another message is to avoid bush meat and contact with bats, since "spillover events," or transmission from animals to people, in Africa have been documented through these sources.

Many challenges remain. While we do know how to stop Ebola through meticulous case finding, isolation, and contact tracing, there is currently no cure or vaccine shown to be safe or effective for Ebola. We are working to strengthen the global response, which requires close collaboration with the World Health Organization (WHO) and additional assistance from our international partners. At CDC, we activated our Emergency Operations Center to respond to the initial outbreak, and are surging our response. As of last week, CDC has over 139 staff in West Africa, and over 1,000 staff in total have provided logistics, staffing, communication, analytics, management, and other support functions. CDC will continue to work with our partners across the United States Government and elsewhere to focus on key strategies of response:

- Effective incident management – CDC is supporting countries to establish national and sub-national Emergency Operations Centers (EOCs) by providing technical assistance and standard operating procedures and embedding staff with expertise in emergency operations. All three West African countries at the center of the epidemic have now named and empowered an Incident Manager to lead efforts.
- Isolation and treatment facilities – It is imperative that we ramp up our efforts to provide adequate space to treat the number of people afflicted with this virus.
- Safe burial practices – Addressing local norms on burial practices is one of the keys to stopping this epidemic. CDC is providing technical assistance for safe burials.
- Infection control throughout the health care system– Good infection control will greatly reduce the spread of Ebola and help control future outbreaks. CDC has a lead role in infection control training for health care workers and safe patient triage throughout the health care system.
- Communications – CDC will continue to effectively communicate facts about the disease and how to contain it, particularly targeting communities in these countries that have presented challenges to date.

The public health response to Ebola rests on the same proven public health approaches that we employ for other outbreaks, and many of our experts are working in the affected countries to rapidly apply these approaches and build local capacity. These include strong surveillance and epidemiology, using real-time data to improve rapid response; case-finding and tracing of the contacts of Ebola patients to identify those with symptoms and monitor their status; and strong laboratory networks that allow rapid diagnosis.

The resources provided for the period of the Continuing Resolution will support our response for the 11 week period of the Continuing Resolution and allow us to ramp up efforts to contain the spread of this virus. More than half of the funds are expected to directly support staff, travel, security and related expenses. A portion of the funds will be provided to the affected area to assist with basic public health infrastructure, such as laboratory and surveillance capacity, and improvements in outbreak management and infection control. The remaining funds will be used for other aspects of strengthening the public health response such as laboratory supplies/equipment, and other urgent needs to enable a rapid and flexible response to an unprecedented global epidemic. CDC is working to identify our resource needs for the rest of the fiscal year, and possibly further, as we deal with this evolving situation. CDC will continue to coordinate activities directly with critical Federal partners—including the United States Agency for International Development (USAID), DoD, DHS, and the State Department—and nongovernmental organizations. Over the past few weeks, we have seen progress, as the DoD has begun deploying assets to the area and laying the ground work to construct 17 ETUs, train local workers to staff these facilities, and move supplies into the area. In addition, USAID is working closely with nongovernmental organizations to scale up efforts in all areas of the response. Currently, there are over 60 burial teams in all 15 counties of Liberia for the management of safe human remains. More than 70 organizations are providing Ebola education and awareness in Liberia, Guinea, and Sierra Leone. Organizations are also working to improve infection control practices in all health facilities to ensure functionality of the healthcare system. We continue to work with national governments, WHO, and USAID to provide for interim measures such as isolation in community settings with proper protections, and improvements to ensure the safe burial of those who have died from the virus.

Though the most effective step we can take to protect the United States is to stop the epidemic where it is occurring, we are also taking strong steps to protect Americans here at home. The imported case of Ebola in Dallas, diagnosed on September 30th in a traveler from Liberia, required CDC and the Nation's public health system to implement rapid response protocols that have been developed in anticipation of such an event. Within hours of confirming that the patient had Ebola, CDC had a team of 10 people on the ground in

Dallas to assist the capable teams from the Texas state health department and local authorities. We have worked side-by-side with state and local officials to do all we can to prevent transmission to others. Together, we assessed all 114 individuals who might possibly have had contact with the patient prior to his admission and isolation. We narrowed down the contacts to 10 who may have been around him when he was infectious and 38 others with whom exposure cannot be ruled out. These individuals will be tracked for 21 days for any signs of symptoms, and they will quickly be isolated if symptoms develop. We are also working to identify and learn lessons from the initial patient encounter and other events that complicated our response, and to apply them in any other responses.

We were deeply concerned to have learned last weekend that there had been transmission of the Ebola virus from the first, or "index" patient, to a health care worker. This health care worker had been monitoring her temperature and symptoms, in accordance with CDC guidelines, and upon finding an elevated temperature, immediately reported it to the hospital and was admitted and isolated. And just yesterday, we learned of a second transmission in another health care worker. While we do not yet know exactly how these transmissions occurred, they demonstrate the need to strengthen the procedures for infection-control protocols which allowed for exposure to the virus. We are working very hard to investigate the situation, but are not waiting for the completion of this investigation and have already helped the hospital implement new measures for safety.

In terms of safe and effective care of Ebola patients, we had already begun to increase education and training of health care workers at the facility which cared for the index patient. The care of Ebola can be done safely, but it requires meticulous and scrupulous attention to infection control, and even a single inadvertent slip can result in contamination. At this time, we are recommending to the facility that the number of workers who care for anyone with suspected Ebola be kept to an absolute minimum. We recommend that the procedures that are undertaken to support the care of an infected individual be limited solely to essential procedures. We are examining the issue of personal protective equipment, understanding that there is a balance and putting more on isn't always safer as it may make it harder to provide effective care. And we are recommending there be a full time individual who is responsible only for the oversight, supervision, and monitoring of effective infection control while an Ebola patient is cared for. Each day we work to evaluate and improve infection control, and these represent measures put into place so far. CDC has sent additional staff to Texas to assist with this response and we will continue to work closely with the State and local team. In particular, we are closely monitoring other health care workers who were part of the care team, because we now have reason to believe had an elevated risk of exposure.

Despite these latest incidents, we remain confident that our public health and health care systems can prevent an Ebola outbreak here, and that the authorities and investments provided by the Congress have put us in a strong position to protect Americans. To make sure the United States is prepared, as the epidemic in West Africa has intensified, CDC has done the following:

- Instituted layers of protection, starting in affected countries where our staff work intensively on airport exit screening, such as temperature scanning for outbound passengers.
- Provided guidance for airline personnel and for DHS U.S. Customs and Border Protection Officers on how to identify sick passengers and how to manage them. Though it was one of many false alarms, the recent incident with an inbound passenger to Newark, New Jersey shows how CDC's quarantine station at the airport worked with airline, DHS, airport, EMS, and hospital personnel to assess and manage a sick passenger, and to protect other passengers and the public.
- Developed guidance for monitoring and movement of people with possible exposures.
- Along with partners in DHS and state and local health agencies, continually assessed and improved approaches to inbound passenger screening and management, and as the President announced on October 6th, CDC is working with DHS to enhance screening measures at United States airports.
- Worked with American hospitals to reinforce and strengthen infection controls, and CDC has provided checklists and instructions to health care facilities to assess patients for travel history. We have also worked with state and local health departments to ensure that these practices are being followed.
- With state health departments, intensified training and outreach to build awareness since the Dallas case.
- Through the Laboratory Response Network (LRN), expanded lab capacity across the United States – in addition to CDC's own world class laboratories, 14 LRN labs now have capacity for testing,

ensuring that we have access to labs for timely assessment – and surge capacity in case it is needed.

- Developed response protocols for the evaluation, isolation, and investigation of any incoming individuals with relevant symptoms.
- Extensively consulted to support evaluation and, when indicated, tested suspect cases. With heightened alert, we are receiving hundreds of inquiries for help in ruling out Ebola in travelers – a sign of how seriously airlines, border agents, and health care system workers are taking this situation. So far just over a dozen of these hundreds of suspect cases have required testing, and only one (the Dallas patient) has been positive.

Our top priority at CDC is to protect Americans from threats. We work 24/7 to do that. In the case of Ebola, we are doing that in many different ways here at home, but we also need to retain our focus on stopping the outbreak at its source, in Africa.

Working with our partners, we have been able to stop every prior Ebola outbreak, and we will stop this one. It will take meticulous work and we cannot take short cuts. It's like fighting a forest fire: leave behind one burning ember, one case undetected, and the epidemic could re-ignite. For example, in response to the case in Nigeria, 10 CDC staff and 40 top CDC-trained Nigerian epidemiologists rapidly deployed, identified, and followed 1,000 contacts for 21 days. Even with these resources, one case was missed, which resulted in a new cluster of cases in Port Harcourt, Nigeria. However, due to the meticulous work done in Nigeria, no new cases have been identified, and the outbreak appears to have been extinguished there.

Ending this epidemic will take time and continued, intensive effort. Before this outbreak began, we had proposed, in the FY 2015 President's Budget, an increase of $45 million to strengthen lab networks that can rapidly diagnose Ebola and other threats, emergency operations centers that can swing into action at a moment's notice, and trained disease detectives who can find an emerging threat and stop it quickly. Building these capabilities around the globe is key to preventing this type of event elsewhere and ensuring countries are prepared to deal with the consequences of outbreaks in other countries. We must do more, and do it quickly, to strengthen global health security around the world, because we are all connected. Diseases can be unpredictable – such as H1N1 coming from Mexico, MERS emerging from the Middle East, or Ebola in West Africa, where it had never been recognized before – which is why we have to be prepared globally for anything nature can create that could threaten our global health security.

Investments in strengthening health systems in West Africa have been very challenging due to the low capacity of the systems. Strengthening the public health infrastructure in West Africa could detect such outbreaks earlier and contain them. This Ebola epidemic shows that any vulnerability could have widespread impact if not stopped at the source.

In February, the United States Government joined with partner governments, WHO and other multilateral organizations, and non-governmental actors to launch the Global Health Security Agenda (GHSA). Over the next five years, the United States has committed to working with over forty partner countries (with a combined population of at least four billion people) to improve their ability to prevent, detect, and effectively respond to infectious disease threats - whether naturally occurring or caused by accidental or intentional release of pathogens. As part of this Agenda, the President's FY 2015 Budget includes $45 million for CDC to accelerate progress in detection, prevention, and response, and we appreciate your support for this investment. We are working to evaluate the needs to strengthen the Ebola-affected nations and neighboring ones most at risk, and are asking that GHSA partners make specific commitments to establish capacity in West African countries in two or three years to prevent, detect and rapidly respond to infectious disease threats. The economic cost of large public health emergencies can be tremendous – the 2003 Severe Acute Respiratory Syndrome epidemic, known as SARS, disrupted travel, trade, and the workplace and cost the Asia-Pacific region alone more than $40 billion. Resources provided for the Global Health Security Agenda can improve detection, prevention, and response and can potentially reduce some of the direct and indirect costs of infectious diseases.

Improving these capabilities for each nation improves health security for all nations. Stopping outbreaks where they occur is the most effective and least expensive way to protect people's health. While this tragic epidemic reminds us that there is still much to be done, we know that sustained commitment and the application of the best evidence and practices will lead us to a safer, healthier world. With a focused effort, and increased vigilance at home, we can stop this epidemic, protect Americans, and leave behind a strong system in West Africa and elsewhere to prevent Ebola and other health threats in the future.

Thank you again for the opportunity to appear before you today. I appreciate your attention to this epidemic and I look forward to answering your questions.

In: Ebola
Editor: MaryAnn Cole
ISBN: 978-1-63482-253-4


*Chapter 5*

# TESTIMONY OF DR. ANTHONY S. FAUCI, DIRECTOR, NATIONAL INSTITUTE OF ALLERGY AND INFECTIOUS DISEASES. HEARING ON "EXAMINING THE U.S. PUBLIC HEALTH RESPONSE TO THE EBOLA OUTBREAK"*

Mr. Chairman, Ranking Member DeGette, and Members of the Subcommittee:

Thank you for the opportunity to discuss the National Institutes of Health (NIH) response to the global health emergency of Ebola virus disease. I direct the National Institute of Allergy and Infectious Diseases (NIAID), the lead institute of the NIH for conducting and supporting research on infectious diseases, including viral hemorrhagic fevers such as those caused by Ebola virus infection.

For over six decades, NIAID has made important contributions to advancing the understanding of infectious, immunologic, and allergic diseases, from basic research on mechanisms of disease to applied research to develop diagnostics, therapeutics, and vaccines. NIAID has a dual mandate that balances research addressing current biomedical challenges with the capacity

* This is an edited, reformatted and augmented version of testimony presented October 16, 2014 before the House Energy and Commerce Committee, Subcommittee on Oversight and Investigations.

to respond quickly to newly emerging and re-emerging infectious diseases, including bioterror threats. Critical to these efforts are NIAID's partnerships with academia, pharmaceutical companies, international organizations such as the World Health Organization (WHO), and collaborations with other Federal entities, particularly the Centers for Disease Control and Prevention, the Food and Drug Administration (FDA), the Biomedical Advanced Research and Development Authority (BARDA), and the Department of Defense (DOD).

## Overview of Ebola Virus Disease

Viral hemorrhagic fevers are severe illnesses that can be fatal and are caused by a diverse group of viruses including Marburg virus, Lassa virus, and Ebola virus. Infection with Ebola virus typically causes fever, severe vomiting, diarrhea, rash, profound weakness, electrolyte loss, impaired kidney and liver function, and in some cases internal and external bleeding. Since the discovery of Ebola virus in 1976, outbreaks of hemorrhagic fever caused by Ebola virus have had fatality rates ranging from 25 percent to 90 percent, depending on the species of virus and the availability of medical facilities and staff to care for infected patients. West Africa is currently experiencing the most severe Ebola outbreak ever recorded. As of October 12, 2014, there have been 8,997 reported cases, including 4,493 documented deaths according to the WHO. The ongoing Ebola epidemic in Guinea, Liberia, and Sierra Leone has generated more cases and deaths than the 24 previous Ebola outbreaks combined. The recent death of a patient diagnosed with Ebola in Dallas, Texas, after traveling from Liberia, and the cases transmitted outside of Africa (to two healthcare workers in Dallas and a nurse in Spain) intensify our concerns about this global health threat.

The ongoing public health crisis in West Africa demands a major amplification of efforts to identify and isolate infected individuals, perform contact tracing, and provide personal protective equipment for healthcare workers involved in the treatment of infected individuals. This still remains the time-proven approach to controlling and ultimately ending the epidemic. However, there is also a critical need to develop improved diagnostics, as well as safe and effective therapeutics and vaccines for Ebola since there are no such FDA-approved interventions available at this time. In this regard, NIAID has a longstanding commitment to advancing research to combat Ebola while ensuring the safety and efficacy of potential medical countermeasures such as treatments and vaccines.

## HISTORY OF NIAID EBOLA VIRUS RESEARCH: RELATIONSHIP TO BIODEFENSE RESEARCH

The ability to safely and effectively prevent and treat Ebola virus infection is a longstanding NIAID priority. Since the 2001 anthrax attacks, NIAID has vastly expanded its research portfolio in biodefense and naturally emerging and re-emerging infectious diseases. This research targets pathogens that pose high risks to public health and national security. NIAID has designated pathogens with high mortality such as anthrax, plague, smallpox, and Ebola virus as NIAID Category A Priority Pathogens to highlight the need for medical countermeasures against these dangerous microbes.

NIAID's expanded research efforts in biodefense and emerging and re-emerging infectious diseases focus on specific objectives. The first is to advance basic and translational research and facilitate development of effective products to combat deadly diseases such as Ebola. The second is to employ innovative strategies, such as broad spectrum vaccines and therapeutics, to prevent and treat a variety of related infectious diseases. The third is to strengthen our partnerships with biotechnology and pharmaceutical companies to help accelerate the availability of needed products for affected and at-risk individuals.

Since 2001, NIAID's biodefense research has supported the development and testing of numerous candidate products to prevent or treat viral hemorrhagic fevers, including those caused by Ebola and other related viruses. The progress we have made with candidate vaccines, therapeutics, and diagnostics for Ebola virus would not be possible had we not made this important investment.

## DEVELOPMENT AND TESTING OF EBOLA MEDICAL COUNTERMEASURES

In response to the Ebola public health emergency in West Africa, NIAID is accelerating ongoing research efforts and partnering with governments and private companies throughout the world to speed the development of medical countermeasures that could help control the current epidemic and future outbreaks. NIAID research on Ebola virus focuses on basic research to understand how Ebola virus causes illness in animals and in people, as well as applied research to develop diagnostics, vaccines, and therapeutics.

## Diagnostics

Accurate and accessible diagnostics for Ebola virus infection are needed for the rapid identification and treatment of patients in an outbreak because the symptoms of Ebola can be easily mistaken for other common causes of fever in affected areas, such as malaria. NIAID continues to provide resources to investigators attempting to develop Ebola diagnostics. With NIAID support, Corgenix Medical Corporation is developing rapid immunodiagnostics for Ebola viruses using genomic technology to produce recombinant viral proteins. NIAID also is advancing development of other types of diagnostics, including those using novel technologies such as microfluidics, optofluidics and nanophotonics, which are capable of detecting an array of viruses including Ebola. Such innovative approaches can provide information critical to the creation of point-of-care diagnostics that could be distributed and used in areas where Ebola virus outbreaks occur. Intramural scientists from NIAID's Rocky Mountain Laboratories (RML) in Hamilton, Montana, and the Integrated Research Facility in Frederick, Maryland, have responded to the epidemic by providing technical diagnostic support on the ground in Liberia.

## Therapeutics

Currently, supportive care, including careful attention to fluid and electrolyte replacement, is the only effective medical intervention for patients with Ebola virus disease; no drugs are available that have been shown safe and effective specifically to treat Ebola virus infection. Experts are now evaluating whether drugs licensed or approved for the treatment of other diseases should be reevaluated for potential treatment of patients with Ebola in the current epidemic on an emergency basis. In parallel, NIAID is supporting the development of novel therapeutics targeting Ebola virus. These investigational candidate therapeutics could possibly be used in clinical trials in the current epidemic and hopefully will prove to be safe and effective; if so, such treatments could be more widely available for future outbreaks. It is important to note that NIAID-supported candidate therapeutics are in early development and are currently available only in limited quantities.

NIAID has provided support to and collaborated with Mapp Biopharmaceutical, Inc., to develop MB-003, a combination of three antibodies that prevents Ebola virus disease in monkeys when administered as late as 48 hours after exposure. An optimized product derived from MB-003, known as ZMapp, has shown to be substantially more effective in animal models than earlier combinations and protected monkeys from death due to Ebola virus up to five days after infection, according to Mapp Biopharmaceutical, Inc. NIAID's preclinical services are now being used to provide pivotal safety data to support the use of ZMapp for clinical trials in humans. Mapp Biopharmaceutical, Inc., has announced that ZMapp was recently administered to humans for the first time as an experimental treatment to several Ebola-infected patients, including two Americans. It is not possible at this time to determine whether ZMapp benefited these patients. NIAID is working closely with partners at DOD, BARDA, and FDA to advance development and testing of ZMapp to determine whether it is safe and effective. BARDA has recently announced plans to optimize and accelerate the manufacturing of ZMapp so that clinical safety testing can proceed as soon as possible.

NIAID also has funded BioCryst Pharmaceuticals to develop and test BCX4430, a novel drug that interferes with the reproductive process of the virus and has activity against a broad spectrum of viruses. According to BioCryst, BCX4430 has protected animals against infection with Ebola virus and the related Marburg virus. BioCryst has announced that a Phase 1 clinical trial of this drug is expected to begin in late 2014 or early 2015. NIAID also is evaluating therapeutics licensed or in development for the treatment of other diseases for their potential activity against Ebola virus. One of these investigational agents is brincidofovir, an antiviral originally developed with NIAID support for use against other viruses.

In related work, NIAID intramural scientists at RML are working on therapeutics that might be effective against all hemorrhagic fever viruses, including the filoviruses Ebola and Marburg and the arenavirus Lassa. Ribavirin, a drug currently used to treat hemorrhagic fever viruses such as Lassa virus, is being examined for its potential use in combination with interferon to treat Ebola virus infection. Other therapeutics are in early stages of study by RML and, if successful, will advance to animal model testing.

## Vaccines

A safe and effective Ebola vaccine could be a critically important tool to help prevent Ebola virus disease and help contain future outbreaks. The hope is that such a vaccine could be licensed and used in the field to protect frontline healthcare workers and individuals living in areas where Ebola virus exists. Two Ebola vaccine candidates are undergoing Phase 1 clinical testing this fall. NIAID will play a critical role in advancing these Ebola vaccine candidates. The results of these Phase 1 studies will inform essential discussions about whether and how such vaccines could be of use in the current epidemic or future Ebola outbreaks.

The NIAID Vaccine Research Center (VRC) has a robust viral hemorrhagic fever vaccine development program. Since 2003, the VRC has evaluated three early-generation Ebola vaccine candidates and one Marburg vaccine candidate in Phase 1 clinical trials at the NIH campus. An additional Phase 1 clinical trial was conducted in Kampala, Uganda, in collaboration with DOD.

None of the early-generation candidates raised safety concerns in these small trials; however, they did not elicit the level of immune response thought to be needed to provide protection against the viruses. The data from those trials have contributed directly to the VRC's current Ebola vaccine collaboration with the pharmaceutical company GlaxoSmithKline (GSK). VRC and GSK have developed an experimental vaccine that uses a chimpanzee virus (similar to the common cold virus), Chimp Adenovirus 3 (CAd3), as a carrier, or vector, to introduce Ebola virus genes into the body; these genes encode Ebola proteins that stimulate an immune response. The vaccine candidate has shown promising results in animal models against two Ebola virus species (bivalent vaccine), including the Zaire Ebola species responsible for the current epidemic in West Africa. A small Phase 1 study to examine the safety and ability of this candidate to induce an immune response in humans began on September 2, 2014, at the NIH Clinical Center in Bethesda, Maryland. All twenty of the study volunteers have been vaccinated. The trial is now moving forward to two other U.S. sites (University of Maryland and Emory University) to gather additional safety and immunogenicity data. Results from all sites are anticipated by the end of 2014 and will inform future development of the vaccine.

As part of Phase 1 studies, the NIH will also support testing of a related vaccine candidate, including just a single Ebola virus gene from the Zaire Ebola virus (monovalent vaccine). NIAID and GSK also have donated doses of this vaccine candidate to enable further testing by NIAID partners in the United Kingdom and the West African country of Mali; the U.K. study has already begun. Plans are underway with GSK and WHO partners for an additional, larger clinical study of the monovalent vaccine in Geneva/Lausanne, Switzerland.

Additionally, starting this month, NIH will collaborate with DOD and NewLink Genetics Corporation on Phase 1 safety studies of an investigational Ebola vaccine based on vesicular stomatitis virus (VSV). The VSV will serve as a vector or carrier for an Ebola gene similar to how the Chimp adenovirus serves as a vector or carrier as described above for the NIAID/GSK vaccine. This vaccine candidate was developed by and licensed from the Public Health Agency of Canada.

In addition to these Ebola candidates entering Phase 1 trials in 2014, NIAID supports a broad portfolio of Ebola vaccine research. NIAID has supported the biopharmaceutical company Crucell to develop a recombinant adenovirus-vectored Ebola vaccine. In animal studies, this vaccine candidate protected against filovirus infection, including Ebola virus. NIAID has played an instrumental role in the recent announcements by Johnson & Johnson (parent company of Crucell) and Bavarian Nordic that they will collaborate on a two dose (prime-boost) vaccination regimen that will begin Phase 1 testing in 2015.

NIAID intramural scientists are collaborating with Thomas Jefferson University investigators to produce a vaccine candidate based on an existing rabies vaccine. The researchers aim to generate immunity to Ebola, Marburg, and rabies viruses, important diseases in certain regions in Africa. The investigators plan to pursue a version of the vaccine for human and veterinary use, as well as a version for use in African wildlife. The wildlife vaccine could help prevent transmission of Ebola virus from animals to humans. The vaccine candidate for use in humans is undergoing preclinical testing and has demonstrated protection against infection by rabies and Ebola viruses in animal models. NIAID is currently partnering with DOD to produce sufficient quantities of the vaccine candidate to begin clinical testing in 2015. In September, NIH licensed the candidate rabies/Ebola vaccines to Exxell BIO of St. Paul, Minnesota, which aims to advance the products through clinical testing and potential commercialization.

NIAID also is supporting the biotechnology company Profectus BioSciences, Inc., to investigate a second recombinant VSV-vectored vaccine candidate against Ebola and Marburg viruses. Profectus is pursing preclinical testing of the vaccine in preparation for a future Phase 1 clinical trial. Additionally, NIAID is collaborating with the Galveston National Laboratory & Institute for Human Infections and Immunity at the University of Texas Medical Branch at Galveston to further progress made by NIAID intramural scientists on a paramyxovirus-based vaccine against Ebola virus.

Other NIAID-supported efforts include Ebola virus vaccine candidates in early development, such as a DNA vaccine targeting Ebola and Marburg viruses, an adenovirus-5- based intranasal Ebola vaccine, and a combination virus-like particle/DNA vaccine targeting Ebola and Marburg viruses to be delivered by microneedle patch. Knowledge gained through these studies will further the goal of the ultimate deployment of a safe and effective vaccine that will prevent this deadly disease.

NIAID also advances vaccine product development by providing preclinical services such as animal testing to researchers in academia and industry. More than 30 different filovirus vaccine formulations have been evaluated through NIAID's preclinical services since 2011 using animal models and assays that NIAID has developed over many years.

## Clinical Trials to Evaluate Efficacy

It is important to balance the urgency to deploy investigational medical countermeasures in an emergency such as the current Ebola outbreak with the need to ensure the maximal safety and to determine the efficacy of candidate drugs and vaccines for Ebola. We will do this with the strictest attention to safety considerations, established scientific principles, and ethical considerations, and compassion for and realization of the immediate needs of the affected populations. The United States Government, working in partnership with industry, has an established mechanism for testing and reviewing the safety and efficacy of potential medical interventions. Randomized controlled clinical trials remain the "gold standard" for the evaluation of candidate drugs and vaccines because they represent the most efficient way to prove efficacy and lack of an unexpected harmful effect. This is particularly important for vaccines since they are administered to healthy individuals.

NIAID is committed to working with our partners to evaluate candidate drugs and vaccines for safety and efficacy. We are working to generate the evidence to show whether potential interventions are safe and effective to reassure affected communities that we are pursuing the tools needed to prevent and treat this deadly disease. Our partnerships with industry will be critical to move these products expeditiously along the development pipeline into clinical trials. NIAID is currently working to accelerate the vaccines discussed above into Phase 1 clinical trials in healthy volunteers. The data from these trials will help demonstrate whether candidate Ebola vaccines are safe in humans and are capable of generating the desired immune response. Candidate Ebola treatments will be similarly evaluated for safety and markers of potential efficacy. If successful, these candidates will be advanced to further testing in larger numbers of people. As we proceed through clinical testing, we will continue to work with our partners in the FDA to accelerate development of and speed access to the products, while also protecting the safety and rights of study volunteers.

## CONCLUSION

While NIAID is an active participant in the global effort to address the public health emergency occurring in West Africa, it is important to recognize that we are still in the early stages of understanding how infection with the Ebola virus can be treated and prevented. As we continue to expedite research while enforcing high safety and efficacy standards, the implementation of the public health measures already known to contain prior Ebola virus outbreaks and the implementation of treatment strategies such as fluid and electrolyte replacement are essential to preventing additional infections, treating those already infected, protecting health care providers, and ultimately bringing this epidemic to an end. We will continue to work with biopharmaceutical companies and public health agencies throughout the world to develop and distribute medical countermeasures for Ebola virus disease as quickly as possible. NIAID remains committed to fulfilling its dual mandate to balance research on current biomedical challenges with the capability to mobilize a rapid response to newly emerging and reemerging infectious diseases.

In: Ebola
Editor: MaryAnn Cole
ISBN: 978-1-63482-253-4


*Chapter 6*

# STATEMENT OF SYLVIA BURWELL, SECRETARY, U.S. DEPARTMENT OF HEALTH AND HUMAN SERVICES. HEARING ON "U.S. GOVERNMENT RESPONSE: FIGHTING EBOLA AND PROTECTING AMERICA"*

Chairwoman Mikulski, Ranking Member Shelby, Chairman Harkin, Ranking Member Moran, and members of the Committee, thank you for inviting me here today to discuss the Department of Health and Human Services' (HHS) response to the current Ebola epidemic, and our request for emergency funding to invest in these ongoing efforts and further strengthen our response. Since the first cases of Ebola were reported in West Africa in March 2014, the United States has mounted a whole-of-Government response to protect the American people and contain and eliminate the epidemic at its source. At HHS, this response involves close coordination between the Centers for Disease Control and Prevention (CDC), the National Institutes of Health (NIH), the Food and Drug Administration (FDA), the Assistant Secretary for Preparedness and Response (ASPR), the Office of Global Affairs (OGA), and the U.S. Public Health Service Commissioned Corps, among others. I appreciate the opportunity to discuss our role in this critical effort and our request for emergency funding to ensure that resources are available for both the immediate and longer-term to meet the evolving nature of the epidemic.

---

* This is an edited, reformatted and augmented version of a statement presented November 12, 2014 before the Senate Committee on Appropriations.

We believe that we have the right strategy in place, both at home and abroad, to respond to Ebola. Our strategy is designed around four core principles. First, to further strengthen our domestic preparedness. While we may see additional cases in the United States, we are confident that we will limit the number of cases here in the country. Second, to stop the epidemic at its source in West Africa, which is also how we best protect our homeland. Third, to accelerate research and development of vaccines, rapid diagnostics, and therapeutics to combat the disease and prevent future outbreaks. Fourth, to urgently establish what is needed to prevent spread of Ebola and to more broadly prevent, detect and rapidly respond to outbreaks before they become epidemics, through the Global Health Security Agenda.

I want to take a moment to recognize the health care and public health workers who are on the front lines of this response – ensuring that our hospitals and communities here at home are prepared and providing care and assistance for those at the source of the outbreak in West Africa. Unfortunately, Thomas Duncan, a visitor from Liberia, died of Ebola in Dallas on October 8$^{th}$. Thankfully, the two Dallas nurses who provided care for Mr. Duncan and became infected have now been declared Ebola-free, including one who was treated at our own NIH Special Clinical Studies Center. Our thoughts and prayers are with Dr. Craig Spencer, who contracted this disease in West Africa while selflessly providing care for others, and with the hundreds of health care workers who are preparing our hospitals here in the United States and continuing the fight abroad, as well as with the people of Liberia, Sierra Leone, and Guinea who are facing this disease in their homes and communities.

## HHS Response

The Department is requesting $2.43 billion in emergency funding to execute our ongoing Ebola response strategy and see it through effectively. With the funding provided under the Fiscal Year 2015 continuing resolution, the Department has scaled up efforts to prepare public health and health care systems in the United States, accelerate research and development of vaccines and therapeutics, and combat and contain the spread of the virus in West Africa. Actions we have taken to date to further strengthen our readiness and recent developments demonstrate why we must continue to invest in our strategy.

Domestic preparedness is a top priority for this Administration, and we have taken a number of active steps as an Administration and at HHS to further strengthen our readiness. These steps include training and support to enable screening of travelers as they leave countries with widespread transmission of Ebola on their way to the United States; funneling those travelers through one of five airports in the United States with enhanced screening mechanisms; and active post-arrival monitoring of those travelers for the full 21-day incubation period.

A central part of our preparedness here at home is ensuring that hospitals are in a position to manage the early recognition and isolation of a patient with Ebola symptoms and engage public health authorities appropriately. While hospitals throughout the country must be able to recognize and safely isolate a potential Ebola patient, we have worked with a targeted subset of hospitals to further strengthen their readiness to treat patients. As we speak, teams of experts are visiting hospitals that have volunteered to take Ebola patients and are assessing and helping to improve their readiness. At the same time, we are working to ensure that transportation from a screening to a treatment hospital is safe and effective. Patients will be transported in an ambulance or, if needed, a plane – in both cases the measures and protocol put in place are designed to protect the patient and the health care workers. CDC is also working with public health laboratories across the United States to build their capacity to test specimens as quickly as possible. If a case is confirmed, CDC has created dedicated response teams to provide immediate on-site assistance to hospitals, as well as state and local public health officials.

As a Department, we have ramped up outreach to hospitals and front-line health care workers. To date, more than a quarter of a million health care personnel have participated in HHS-sponsored information events. That includes calls with 10,000 nurses, 20,000 physicians and dentists, and targeted outreach to emergency responders, laboratory workers, waste management workers, hospital executives, and others involved at all levels of the response. CDC has also updated infection-prevention protocols for hospitals and health care workers, aircraft crew and airport personnel, and laboratories handling specimens from suspected cases to ensure that personnel take all available and scientifically-based precautions to keep themselves safe.

In addition to the successes at Emory University Hospital, the University of Nebraska Medical Center, and the NIH Special Clinical Studies Center, we are hearing encouraging news from the hospitals that have treated and are preparing to treat Ebola patients here in the United States —from Bellevue in New York, which treated Dr. Spencer to Duke University in North Carolina, which screened a potential patient just last week. Of the nine patients treated in the U.S., eight have survived. We have also seen positive signs about our screening and monitoring system. There have been examples in Oklahoma, North Carolina, Oregon, and Maryland where individuals reported symptoms to local authorities based on the screening and monitoring process. The Maryland case is a good example. When the traveler arrived at JFK from Liberia, she was given a CDC issued "CARE kit" with a thermometer and instructions for whom to contact if she started having symptoms. She took her temperature using the CDC thermometer as directed. When it read high she called the Maryland Heath Department as instructed in the CARE kit and the health department facilitated her arrival at the hospital the state referred her to for evaluation. Fortunately, she tested negative. In this case and each of the others, the response followed protocol, minimizing exposure to the public, and in each of these cases the test results turned out to be negative.

The fact is, the best way to protect Americans here at home is to stop Ebola at the source. We have teams from across the Department on the ground in West Africa working alongside the U.S. embassies, the U.S. Agency for International Development (USAID), the U.S. military, local authorities, and non-governmental organizations. Since the start of the outbreak, CDC has deployed more than 600 people to the region to assist with outbreak control, support laboratory and surveillance capacity, and conduct contact tracing. HHS has also deployed a total of 73 specialized Public Health Service Commissioned Corps officers to Liberia to manage and staff a hospital that was constructed by the Department of Defense (DoD) for health care workers who become ill. We are proud of these brave and dedicated men and women from across the Department, and grateful for their service and sacrifice.

Across HHS our employees are working with partners in the private-sector and around the world to develop vaccines and therapeutics to combat this disease. This work is crucial to our efforts government-wide to prevent future outbreaks, and may be needed to help halt the current epidemic. NIH has accelerated research and early development of Ebola vaccine and therapeutic candidates, which are then transitioned to ASPR's Biomedical Advanced Research and Development Authority (BARDA) for advanced development and manufacturing. BARDA is using funds provided under the continuing resolution to begin manufacturing Ebola vaccine candidates and potential therapeutics that will be used for clinical trials. While efforts to date have been critical, additional resources are necessary to bring safe and effective products to FDA approval.

On a parallel track, FDA is actively working to help expedite the development and availability of medical products – including treatments, vaccines, diagnostic tests, and personal protective equipment – with the potential to help bring the epidemic under control as quickly as possible. In addition, FDA has exercised its Emergency Use Authorization (EUA) authority five separate times to allow the use of Ebola diagnostics tests developed by U.S. Government agencies and private industry for the treatment of patients. I want to thank the Congress for providing that authority, and I believe this is an important example of FDA delivering on an authority provided by the Congress to serve the American people.

## EMERGENCY APPROPRIATIONS REQUEST

Although the U.S. Government's response to the Ebola outbreak to date has resulted in progress, additional funding is needed to plan and execute most effectively. The $2.43 billion emergency request for the Department is designed around three core principles: first, $1.22 billion to further strengthen the Department's ongoing strategy to prepare our public health and health care systems here at home, and to invest in the vaccines and treatments that may be used in responding to the current outbreak and in preventing future outbreaks; second, $603 million to stop the outbreak in West Africa; and third, $606 million to strengthen global health security, which reduces risks to Americans by enhancing capacity for high-priority countries to prevent disease outbreaks, detect them early, and swiftly respond before they become epidemics that threaten our national security. These are the same activities that are necessary to combat the spread of Ebola and reduce the potential for future outbreaks of infectious diseases that could follow a similarly devastating, costly, and destabilizing trajectory.

The emergency request also includes $751 million through a Contingency Fund. Resources provided to HHS through the Contingency Fund would only be made available following a Presidential emergency declaration, consistent with the funding structure used by the Congress in 2009 for the emergency funding for the H1N1 pandemic influenza. Given the changing nature of the Ebola epidemic, the Contingency Fund is requested to ensure that there are resources available to respond to the evolving situation. These funds can be transferred among Federal agencies to help meet any critical needs that may arise rapidly. For example, funds could be provided to the Department of Homeland Security to increase Customs and Border Control operations. If necessary, the Contingency Fund also could support increased domestic efforts, such as a limited vaccination clinical trial campaign that could target health care workers treating infected patients (if a vaccine is proven safe and effective); an expanded response in Guinea and Sierra Leone; and enhanced global health security. As the rapidly evolving and unpredictable outbreak progresses, it will be necessary to have maximum flexibility to respond quickly.

## Domestic Preparedness and Response

The Department will use $787 million of the funds provided through the emergency request to enhance ongoing preparedness and response efforts here in the United States, including by strengthening hospital and public health capacity to identify and respond to potential Ebola cases.

Of this funding, $621 million will support CDC's ongoing efforts to ensure that states and localities across the United States have the resources they need to prevent, detect, and respond to Ebola. The funding will strengthen public health and health care systems by improving readiness in hospitals, laboratories and communities across the country. With this funding, CDC will also support state and local health departments in their efforts to improve safety practices of their clinical laboratories and accelerate infection control implementation throughout U.S. hospitals. This includes hiring additional Career Epidemiology Field Officers to conduct contact investigation and monitoring for suspected cases, among other functions. It will also allow CDC to accelerate the development of training courses, materials and videos; work with local hospitals and public health departments to conduct exercises and develop improvement plans; and purchase additional personal protective equipment to be used as needed. Lastly, CDC will continue to work with Federal, state, international, and private partners to ensure proper protocols are followed to identify and quarantine any travelers with a suspected case of Ebola, including enhanced entrance screening, contact tracing and monitoring of suspected cases.

In coordination with CDC's efforts, $166 million is for ASPR to work to strengthen domestic preparedness efforts through improved hospital infrastructure, resources, and training. To optimize efficiency and communication in these efforts, ASPR will utilize its existing Hospital Preparedness Program infrastructure, which provides leadership and funding to states, territories, and eligible municipalities to improve surge capacity and enhance community and hospital preparedness for public health emergencies. The requested funding will support the renovation and alteration of treatment hospitals designated to provide definitive care for patients diagnosed with or suspected to have Ebola. ASPR will also provide funding to states to support the purchase of personal protective equipment and the training of thousands of other hospitals so that their staff can screen for, identify, and provide initial care for Ebola patients. This funding will support giving hospitals and health care workers the training and equipment they need to properly care for Ebola patients while maintaining their own safety.

## INTERNATIONAL RESPONSE

In West Africa, we are optimistic that our strategy is starting to have an impact, with declines in the number of new cases in parts of Liberia. However, progress is fragile and fluid, the number of new cases in Sierra Leone is still growing, hot spots continue in rural, remote parts of Guinea and Liberia, and more work needs to be done, especially to scale up. From the emergency request, HHS will use $603 million to continue to contribute to the whole-of-Government public health response on the international scale, with a focus on long-term system transformation to identify and prevent the spread of future outbreaks. CDC will focus on enhancing infection control and contact tracing; training public health workers both before deployment and in Africa; strengthening laboratory systems and the establishment of national and regional networks; enhancing public health education and outreach for health care workers; procuring and managing in-country operations and supplies for CDC responders during deployment; and establishing Emergency Operations Centers to analyze, validate, and efficiently work with emergency response partners to make sure they have the information and resources they need to operate effectively on the ground. Collectively, this means that we will be better positioned to rapidly diagnose, report and track Ebola cases in the affected countries, that our health care workers on the frontline of this response will be most effectively prepared for their work on the ground, and that we will be able to limit the spread of infection within the health care and community setting.

The Department will continue to work with communities, governments and other partners on the ground in West Africa to ensure that people are promptly diagnosed, effectively treated and, if they die, safely buried. While progress is fluid due to the evolving nature of the epidemic, to date these tactics do appear to be having an impact.

## VACCINES, THERAPEUTICS, AND DIAGNOSTICS

On a separate track, HHS's science agencies will use $420 million of the funding requested to invest in research and development of vaccines, therapeutics, and diagnostics to combat the virus. Of this amount, $238 million is for the NIH National Institute of Allergy and Infectious Diseases (NIAID), home to the doctors and other health care workers who provided care for one of the Dallas nurses who recovered from the virus, to support new and accelerated research to diagnose, treat, and prevent Ebola. In addition to NIAID's treatment capabilities for Ebola patients, much of the requested funding will support clinical trials to evaluate the safety and efficacy of investigational vaccines and therapeutics. This request will also support pre-clinical testing and discovery of new vaccines, therapeutics, and diagnostics to accelerate initial identification and evaluation of their toxicity, immunogenicity, and efficacy. Candidates that show notable progress within this early development could be transitioned into a pipeline of products for advanced development and manufacturing at ASPR/BARDA. Many of these activities could yield initial results in less than a year.

Within ASPR/BARDA, $157 million in additional funding will support the manufacture of vaccines and other therapeutics for use in clinical trials. The funding will also support advanced development for new antibody and therapeutic options, which are available due to successful early development at NIH. This request will support the continued and timely manufacturing and development of antibody products, therapeutics, and vaccine candidates into FY 2016. It also will allow the Federal Government to continue the acceleration of these products towards FDA approval.

The request also includes $25 million for FDA to sustain its aggressive efforts to support the pipeline of possible investigational medical products for Ebola and other serious emerging infectious diseases, including accelerating product development and review, facilitating access to investigational products, and supporting product surveillance. The funding will allow FDA to bring on additional staff to support the Ebola response by providing regulatory and scientific guidance and conducting product review, among other functions, to help expedite the availability of medical products for Ebola. This funding will also enable FDA to conduct the regulatory science research necessary to facilitate the development and regulatory review of such products with the speed required.

## Global Health Security

With an eye towards detecting and preventing outbreaks of this magnitude in the future, the emergency request includes $606 million to urgently strengthen global health security in high-priority countries around the world. The most effective way to prevent the spread of disease to the United States is to address it immediately at its source. This requires building and strengthening critical health infrastructures in countries that are particularly susceptible to Ebola virus disease importation and outbreaks of other high impact infectious disease – meaning strengthening safe and secure laboratory capability to find diseases when they occur, standing up emergency operations centers, providing equipment and training to test patients and report data in real-time, and training the disease detectives needed to track the response. These activities are necessary to combat the spread of Ebola but also to reduce the potential for future outbreaks of infectious diseases that could follow a similarly devastating, costly, and destabilizing trajectory. More specifically, we will make it a priority to focus on countries in the ring around Guinea, Liberia and Sierra Leone, others in the region that are high-priority due to poor infrastructure and countries serving as major air transport hubs with the three affected countries.

Expediting the capability required to prevent, detect and rapidly respond to outbreaks before they become epidemics that threaten the American people is a top priority for HHS and the Administration. The Ebola epidemic, as well as other outbreaks of continuing concern, such as the Middle East Respiratory Syndrome Coronavirus in the Middle East and Ebola in West Africa, underscore that, in a world as interconnected as ours, outbreaks anywhere in the world are a threat to the United States and our global partners. Over the past decade, infectious disease outbreaks have sown fear, cost lives and been a drain on the global economy. For example, the Severe Acute Respiratory Syndrome cost the global economy an estimated $40 billion. During the anthrax attacks of 2001, 22 people were infected, five people lost their lives here in in the United States, and the cleanup cost was more than a billion dollars. The global H1N1 influenza pandemic of 2009 killed 284,000 people worldwide in its first year alone. To contain threats at the source, before they threaten global security, we must immediately invest in shoring up capability in the highest-priority nations.

## Conclusion

The Congress is a key partner in the response to the Ebola epidemic, and I appreciate the attention that you and your colleagues have paid to this important issue. I look forward to working with you on our response and ensuring that HHS and our partners have the necessary resources not only to control and eliminate this epidemic, but also to make the investments necessary to protect us from similar outbreaks going forward. We are committed to protecting the health and safety of the American people and contributing to the worldwide response.

Thank you for the opportunity to testify. I would be happy to answer any questions you may have.

In: Ebola
Editor: MaryAnn Cole
ISBN: 978-1-63482-253-4


*Chapter 7*

# STATEMENT OF JEH JOHNSON, SECRETARY, U.S. DEPARTMENT OF HOMELAND SECURITY. HEARING ON "U.S. GOVERNMENT RESPONSE: FIGHTING EBOLA AND PROTECTING AMERICA"*

Chairwoman Mikulski, Ranking Member Shelby, and Members of this Committee, thank you for the opportunity to testify today about the role and responsibility of the Department of Homeland Security in our Government's response to the Ebola outbreak in West Africa.

DHS is committed to taking every necessary and appropriate step to ensure that the traveling public and the American people are safe. We have already taken a number of important and targeted actions to provide additional layers of protection to the protocols we already have in place to minimize the risk of Ebola in the United States.

DHS, through authorities implemented by the Transportation Security Administration (TSA) and U.S. Customs and Border Protection (CBP), will deny boarding to passengers whom the Centers for Disease Control and Prevention (CDC) or other appropriate medical authority have identified as potentially having a communicable disease, presenting a threat to public health, and should be prevented from traveling via commercial aircraft. We

---

* This is an edited, reformatted and augmented version of a statement presented November 12, 2014 before the Senate Committee on Appropriations.

have in fact used this authority to deny boarding to prevent the spread of Ebola.

In the three affected countries Liberia, Sierra Leone and Guinea local authorities have themselves put in place enhanced screening of air passengers before they leave the country. The CDC is assisting with exit screening and communications in West Africa to prevent sick travelers from boarding planes.

It is my understanding that this enhanced screening has prevented a number of people who may have Ebola from leaving the country.

CDC has also issued guidance about Ebola virus infection for airline flight crews and cleaning and cargo personnel.

At present, there are no direct flights from Liberia, Sierra Leone and Guinea to the United States. To fly here, a commercial air traveler must transit in one of several airports, mostly in Europe. A number of these countries at which transit airports are located specifically Belgium, Canada, France, Germany, the Netherlands and the United Kingdom have also instituted enhanced screening of passengers arriving from the three affected countries.

Upon arrival into the United States, CBP routinely screen passengers for communicable diseases before they are admitted. In doing so, CBP officers observe all passengers arriving in the United States for overt signs of illness and, as appropriate, question travelers at all U.S. ports of entry. When a traveler exhibits overt signs of illness, CBP coordinates with the CDC and public health authorities to immediately assess the medical condition of the traveler.

When notified of an ill traveler prior to the arrival of a flight, CBP, CDC and other first responder personnel meet the flight and conduct a medical evaluation on board the aircraft. For situations identified within the port of entry, the assessment is conducted within designated areas that afford a safe environment for everyone.

At my direction, we have instituted enhanced screening measures at five U.S. international airports that have received about 94 percent of air passengers from Liberia, Sierra Leone, and Guinea, to augment the procedures already in place. The five airports are New York John F. Kennedy, Newark Liberty, Chicago O'Hare, Washington Dulles and Hartsfield-Jackson Atlanta. We began this enhanced screening at JFK Airport on October 11 and at the remaining four airports on October 16.

At these five airports, travelers from the affected countries undergo enhanced screening measures consisting of targeted questions and a temperature check, through the use of non-contact thermal thermometers. The object is to determine whether the passengers are experiencing symptoms or may have been exposed to Ebola. Detailed contact information is also collected in the event the CDC needs to contact them in the future. If there is reason to believe a passenger has been exposed to Ebola, either through the questionnaire, temperature check, or overt symptoms, the passenger will be referred to tertiary screening in a separate area where CDC personnel conduct an evaluation. The CDC has surged staff to these airports to support this mission requirement.

To provide greater efficiency and centralization of our efforts at these airports, we took an additional step on October 22, in cooperation with the airlines and industry partners. At that time, DHS began directing airlines flying passengers who originated in one of the three affected countries to make first entry into the United States at one of the five airports with enhanced screening. This step ensures that 100 percent of travelers who are identified as flying to the United States from the affected countries are screened with these enhanced measures.

If an air traveler wants to fly today to the United States from Liberia, Sierra Leone, or Guinea, the airlines will not permit the passenger to fly on a connecting flight to any U.S. airport other than one of the five with the enhanced screening. We recognize the inconvenience this may cause the few air travelers from West Africa not already scheduled to land at one of these five airports, but we believe this is a necessary and appropriate part of our layered approach to security and the protection of the American people.

So, what we have is that at every point from the port of origin to the port of entry and ports in between air travelers from Liberia, Sierra Leone and Guinea to the United States are being screened.

In addition to these added screening measures, DHS has also done the following:

CBP and TSA have posted messages from the CDC in appropriate languages at selected airport locations that provide awareness on how to prevent the spread of infectious disease, typical symptoms of Ebola, health signs to look for, and information for their doctors should they need to seek medical attention in the future.

CBP officers are also asking all passengers traveling on a passport from Liberia, Sierra Leone, and Guinea, regardless of where they traveled from, whether they have been in one of the three countries in the prior 21 days. If the traveler has been in one of the three countries in the prior 21 days, he or she will be referred for additional screening and, if necessary, CDC or other medical personnel in the area will be contacted pursuant to existing protocols.

All CBP officers are trained to identify the characteristics of potentially infected travelers and to employ CDC-developed protocols that assume every direct contact with body fluids is infectious. CBP also pre-positions protective equipment and safety supplies at all ports of entry and other locations where officers come into contact with the public.

The Coast Guard is also taking a proactive role to protect our seaports. Before any vessel docks at a U.S. port, vessel operators are required to provide advance information about the vessel's last five ports of call, crew and passenger manifests, embarkation ports of crewmembers, and hazardous conditions to include any illness aboard. In consultation with the CDC, the Coast Guard is authorized to restrict a vessel's movement and prohibit entry into U.S. waters should there be concern about an individual with a communicable disease on board.

We are continually evaluating whether additional travel restrictions or screening and precautionary measures are necessary to protect the American people, and I will not hesitate to take any and all appropriate steps to protect the American public.

The projected cost for this Department's Ebola response activities in Fiscal Year 2015 is $13.2 million. The majority of the cost, $10.2 million, is for the enhanced medical screening personnel contract. The remainder is for personal protective equipment, overtime, and other support costs associated with the Department's response. At this point, the Department can manage these requirements within our Fiscal Year 2015 resources.

In closing, I would like to thank all our CBP and TSA officers, the Coast Guard, and other DHS personnel for their dedication to the Department's response to this challenge. I have spoken to them, and visited with them, and I am constantly impressed by their professionalism and commitment to duty. They set a calm and reassuring example for all of us.

Thank you for listening and I look forward to your questions.

In: Ebola
Editor: MaryAnn Cole

ISBN: 978-1-63482-253-4


*Chapter 8*

# EBOLA: SELECTED LEGAL ISSUES*

***Jared P. Cole, Rodney M. Perry, Alissa M. Dolan, Jon O. Shimabukuro, Michael John Garcia, Jane M. Smith and Edward C. Liu***

## SUMMARY

Several West African countries are currently grappling with an unprecedented outbreak of Ebola virus disease (EVD). Here in the United States, where Ebola is not endemic, a handful of EVD cases have been diagnosed, and domestic transmission of the virus has occurred in only two cases to date. This report provides a brief overview of selected legal issues regarding measures to prevent transmission of Ebola virus and the civil rights of individuals affected by the disease.

Quarantine and isolation are restrictions on a person's movement, imposed to prevent the spread of contagious disease. The federal government has jurisdiction over interstate and border quarantine, carried out by the Centers for Disease Control and Prevention (CDC). However, primary quarantine authority typically resides with state health departments and health officials. Every state has the authority to pass and enforce quarantine laws as an exercise of its police powers, but these laws may vary widely by state. State and federal quarantine or isolation orders may be subject to suits alleging inadequate due process or violations of

---

* This is an edited, reformatted and augmented version of a Congressional Research Service publication R43829, prepared for Members and Committees of Congress, dated December 16, 2014.

equal protection, but modern legal challenges to quarantine and isolation orders are not extensive.

In addition to the quarantine and isolation of persons within the United States, some have proposed limiting the entry of persons traveling to the United States from countries experiencing high rates of EVD transmission. Federal agencies' authority to restrict or regulate the entry into the United States of persons who are suspected of carrying Ebola virus or other communicable diseases depends largely upon whether the person is a foreign or U.S. national. Aliens who have been determined to carry Ebola virus may be denied entry, but the health-related grounds for exclusion do not apply to most lawful permanent residents who briefly travel abroad. U.S. citizens abroad may enjoy a constitutional right to reenter the country, in which case the government would be required, at a minimum, to overcome a heavier burden to justify a reentry restriction.

Proposals to restrict air travel to and from affected countries—regardless of citizenship—have also been discussed. The Federal Aviation Administration (FAA) has acknowledged its authority to restrict the use of U.S. airspace, but has cautioned that decisions made on a public health basis would involve other federal agencies. Additionally, the Do Not Board (DNB) list provides a mechanism for U.S. and international health officials to request that specific persons be restricted from boarding commercial aircraft to the United States, on the basis that those persons present a public health risk. Independently, airlines may reserve the right to deny transportation to passengers who may pose a safety risk, but must act consistent with federal nondiscrimination laws.

The use of these measures to contain the spread of Ebola may raise a classic civil rights issue: to what extent can an individual's liberty be curtailed to advance the common good? In addition to the constitutional issues noted above, discrimination against individuals with an infectious disease may be covered by Section 504 of the Rehabilitation Act, the Americans with Disabilities Act (ADA), or the Air Carrier Access Act (ACAA). While quarantine and isolation effectively minimize Ebola exposure, they may also raise various employment concerns, particularly for those workers who fear losing their jobs or wages if they are forced to comply with a quarantine or isolation order. Infected workers may also be protected under the Family and Medical Leave Act (FMLA) if it can be established that they have a serious health condition, and employers whose employees could face workplace exposure to Ebola virus may be obligated to comply with applicable Occupational Safety and Health Administration (OSHA) requirements.

# INTRODUCTION

Ebola virus disease (EVD), also known as Ebola hemorrhagic fever, is a deadly communicable disease typically found only in parts of Africa.[1] Once contracted by a human, the virus can be transmitted to others through direct contact with the bodily fluids of an infected individual. An individual who has contracted Ebola virus is not thought to be contagious before symptoms of EVD (such as fever, diarrhea, or vomiting) are observed.

Several West African countries are currently grappling with an unprecedented outbreak of EVD. Here in the United States, where Ebola is not endemic, two undiagnosed EVD cases have been imported from the West African outbreak.[2] In one of these cases, two nurses were infected by the virus while caring for the patient, representing the first instances of Ebola transmission within the United States.[3]

State and federal governments have significant experience dealing with communicable diseases generally, and both levels of government have taken measures to respond to the domestic EVD cases and minimize the further spread of the virus. The federal government has also taken measures to prevent further entry of persons who may have contracted Ebola virus. However, the high fatality rate of EVD may raise questions regarding the sufficiency of state and federal governments' responses to protect against this particular public health threat. Further, the responses to the current Ebola outbreak raise a classic civil rights issue: to what extent can an individual's liberty be curtailed to advance the common good?[4]

In order to help policy makers evaluate these questions, this report provides a brief overview of the scope of state and federal authorities that have been employed, or may be employed in the future, to prevent transmission of Ebola virus, as well as potential limits on these authorities under current law.

# PREVENTING SPREAD OF THE DISEASE

Efforts to prevent further spread of Ebola have focused on restricting the movement of persons who have been exposed to the virus or who are known to have contracted the virus. Actual and proposed measures to accomplish this include using quarantine or isolation orders under federal or state authority, imposing entry restrictions at the U.S. border, and limiting international air travel to the United States.

## Quarantine and Isolation Authority[5]

### *Federal Quarantine Authority*

Although the terms are often used interchangeably, quarantine and isolation are two distinct concepts. Quarantine typically refers to separating or restricting the movement of individuals who have been exposed to a contagious disease but are not sick.[6] Isolation refers to separating infected individuals from those who are not sick.[7] Primary quarantine authority typically resides with state health departments and health officials; however, the federal government has jurisdiction over interstate and border quarantine.

Federal quarantine and isolation authority derives from the Commerce Clause of the U.S. Constitution, which states that Congress shall have the power "[t]o regulate Commerce with foreign Nations, and among the several states."[8] Section 361 of the Public Health Service Act (PHS Act) grants the Secretary of Health and Human Services (Secretary) the authority to make and enforce regulations necessary "to prevent the introduction, transmission, or spread of communicable diseases from foreign countries into the States or possessions, or from one State or possession into any other State or possession."[9] The law provides the Secretary with broad authority to apprehend, detain, or conditionally release a person. However, the Secretary may only exercise this authority in relation to communicable diseases published in an executive order issued by the President.[10] Executive Order 13295[11] lists the communicable diseases for which this quarantine authority may be exercised.[12] In 2000, the Secretary transferred certain authorities related to persons, including quarantine authority, to the Director of the Centers for Disease Control and Prevention (CDC).[13] Both interstate and foreign quarantine measures are now carried out by CDC's Division of Global Migration and Quarantine.[14] The CDC maintains quarantine stations at 20 ports of entry and land-border crossings, including at international airports in the following areas: Atlanta (ATL), Chicago (ORD), Detroit (DTW), Honolulu (HNL), Houston (IAH), Los Angeles (LAX), Miami (MIA), Minneapolis-St. Paul (MSP), New York City (JFK), Philadelphia (PHL), San Francisco (SFO), San Juan (SJU), Seattle (SEA), and Washington, DC (IAD).[15]

Generally, federal regulations authorizing the apprehension, detention, examination, or conditional release of individuals are applicable only to individuals coming into a state or possession from a foreign country or possession.[16] But Section 361 of the PHS Act also authorizes the apprehension and examination of any individual reasonably believed to be infected with a communicable disease in a qualifying stage[17] and

(a) to be moving or about to move from a State to another State; or
(b) to be a probable source of infection to individuals who, while infected with such disease in a qualifying stage, will be moving from a State to another State.[18]

If found to be infected, such individuals may be detained for such time and in such manner as may be reasonably necessary.[19] Regulations promulgated pursuant to quarantine authority under the PHS Act may be found in Parts 70 and 71 of Title 42 of the *Code of Federal Regulations*. Part 70 applies to interstate travel, Part 71 to foreign arrivals.[20]

In addition, the Director of the CDC is also authorized to take measures as may be necessary to prevent the spread of a communicable disease from one state or possession to any other state or possession if he determines that measures taken by local health authorities are inadequate to prevent the spread of the disease.[21] To prevent the spread of diseases between states, the regulations prohibit infected persons from traveling from one state to another without a permit from the health officer of the state, possession, or locality of destination, if such a permit is required under the law applicable to the place of destination.[22]

Section 311 of the PHS Act[23] provides for federal-state cooperative activities to enforce quarantines. The federal government may assist states and localities in enforcing their quarantines and other health regulations and, in turn, may accept state and local assistance in enforcing federal quarantines.

***State Quarantine Authority***

While the federal government has authority to authorize quarantine and isolation under certain circumstances, the primary authority for quarantine and isolation exists at the state level as an exercise of the state's police power. The CDC acknowledges this deference to state authority as follows:

> In general, CDC defers to the state and local health authorities in their primary use of their own separate quarantine powers. Based upon long experience and collaborative working relationships with our state and local partners, CDC continues to anticipate the need to use this federal authority to quarantine an exposed person only in rare situations, such as events at ports of entry or in similar time-sensitive settings.[24]

Although every state has the authority to pass and enforce quarantine laws as an exercise of its police powers, these laws vary widely by state. Generally, state and local quarantines are authorized through public health orders, though some states may require a court order before an individual is detained.[25] For example, in Louisiana, the state health officer is not authorized to "confine [a person] in any institution unless directed or authorized to do so by the judge of the parish in which the person is located."[26] Diseases subject to quarantine may be defined by statute, with some statutes addressing only a single disease, or the state health department may be granted the authority to decide which diseases are communicable and therefore subject to quarantine.[27] States also employ different methods for determining the duration of the quarantine or isolation period. Generally, "release is accomplished when a determination is made that the person is no longer a threat to the public health, or no longer infectious."[28]

Federal authority over interstate and foreign travel is clearly delineated under constitutional and statutory provisions. However, in a public health emergency, federal, state, and local authorities may overlap. For example, both federal and state agencies may have quarantine authority over an aircraft arriving in a large city from a foreign country. Thus, coordination between the various levels of government would be essential during a widespread public health emergency.

### *Legal Challenges to Quarantine*

Constitutional rights to due process and equal protection may be implicated by the imposition of a quarantine or isolation order. Modern legal challenges to quarantine and isolation orders are not extensive, although a few cases can provide some basic insights about potential issues. In 1963, a federal district court in *United States v. Shinnick* upheld the U.S. Public Health Service's medical isolation of an arriving passenger because she had been in Stockholm, Sweden, while the city had been declared by the World Health Organization to be a smallpox-infected area, and she could not show proof of vaccination.[29] The court declined to substitute its own judgment as to whether the plaintiff had been exposed to infection and capable of spreading the disease.

However, at least one state court has ruled that when a state confines an individual in order to prevent the spread of disease, the state must provide the individual with procedural due process protections, such as, *inter alia*, notice explaining the grounds for confinement, the right to counsel, and the right to engage in cross-examination.[30] This requirement would presumably apply to a federal government quarantine order as well. Quarantines may also be subject to equal protection challenges. In *Jew Ho v. Williamson*, for example, a court invalidated a quarantine whose requirements applied only to Chinese residents because it was "unreasonable, unjust and oppressive" and constituted discrimination in violation of the Fourteenth Amendment.[31]

## Border Entry Issues [32]

Federal law confers executive agencies with significant authority to restrict or regulate the entry into the United States of persons who are suspected of carrying Ebola virus or other communicable diseases. However, the stringency of the available restrictions depends upon whether the person is a foreign or U.S. national.

### *Inadmissibility of Infected Aliens*

Foreign nationals do not have a constitutional right to be admitted into the United States.[33] The Immigration and Nationality Act (INA) provides various grounds under which a foreign national may be denied admission, including when he or she is determined to have a "communicable disease of public health significance."[34] The Secretary of the Department of Health and Human Services (HHS) is responsible for defining illnesses constituting a "communicable disease of public health significance" for INA purposes. Current HHS regulations define the term to include diseases, such as EVD, that are listed in a relevant executive order[35] and/or are subject to specified requirements under the rules of the World Health Organization.[36] Accordingly, aliens who have been determined to carry Ebola virus may be denied entry into the United States.[37]

The health-related grounds for exclusion do not apply to most lawful permanent resident aliens (sometimes described as immigrants) who briefly travel abroad.[38] Moreover, assessing whether a foreign national is inadmissible on health-related grounds is an individualized determination of the person's condition, rather than a more general bar applicable to persons who might have had contact with a person carrying a communicable disease. It is also not assured that a foreign national carrying Ebola virus will be identified as such either when applying for a visa to come to the United States (e.g., if the foreign national only became infected after obtaining a visa) or when processed upon arrival at a U.S. port of entry (e.g., if the infected person did not show symptoms of EVD at the time of arrival into the United States).

***Blanket Restrictions on Entry of Travelers from Ebola-Stricken Countries***

Although the government enjoys authority under federal immigration law to bar the entry of many foreign nationals on specific health-related grounds, as noted above, application of these grounds might not be wholly effective in preventing foreign travelers carrying Ebola from being admitted into the United States. Several Members of Congress have gone further and suggested a blanket ban on the admission into the United States of foreign nationals who reside in or have recently traveled to Ebola-stricken countries[39]—a suggestion that the Obama Administration has thus far opposed.[40]

Section 212(f) of the INA provides that the President, pursuant to a proclamation, may direct the denial of entry to any alien or class of aliens whose entry into the country "would be detrimental to the interests of the United States," including potentially those foreign travelers who have already been issued a visa to travel to the United States.[41] Although this provision seems to have never been employed so broadly,[42] it could potentially be used to restrict the entry of foreign nationals traveling from a particular country or region where there has been an Ebola outbreak. If the President deems the entry of such persons into the country to be contrary to U.S. interests, such a restriction would obviate the need to determine if an individual had actually been infected by Ebola virus.

These immigration-related restrictions apply exclusively to foreign nationals, not U.S. citizens. Indeed, U.S. citizens abroad may enjoy a constitutional right to reenter the country, in which case the government would be required, at a minimum, to overcome a heavier burden to justify a reentry restriction than would be required in situations where a person's constitutional rights were not implicated.[43] However, various travel restrictions discussed elsewhere in this report may impede the ability of any person—regardless of citizenship—from traveling to the United States in a manner that potentially exposes others to a communicable disease.[44]

## Airlines and Travel Restrictions[45]

There are currently no scheduled nonstop flights on commercial airlines between the West African countries with widespread Ebola transmission—Guinea, Liberia, and Sierra Leone—and the United States.[46] On average, about 150 passengers travel from the three affected countries to the United States daily.[47] The majority of these passengers travel to the United States via connecting flights in Europe.[48]

On October 21, 2014, the Department of Homeland Security (DHS) announced that all passengers arriving in the United States whose travel originates in one of the affected countries will be required to fly into one of the following airports with enhanced screening procedures in place: John F. Kennedy International Airport (JFK); Newark Liberty International Airport (EWR); Washington Dulles International Airport (IAD); Hartsfield-Jackson Atlanta International Airport (ATL); and Chicago O'Hare International Airport (ORD).[49] Effective November 17, 2014, these restrictions were extended to passengers whose travel originates in Mali, as a precaution in light of a number of new confirmed EVD cases there.[50]

### *Federal Airspace Authority*

The notion that each nation has complete and exclusive sovereignty over the airspace above its territory has been incorporated into international agreements dating back to the initial rise of international aviation.[51] In 1958, Congress enshrined this principle in federal law by declaring that "The United States Government has exclusive sovereignty of airspace of the United States."[52] Congress delegated the authority to regulate U.S. airspace to the administrator of the Federal Aviation Administration (FAA).[53] The FAA has the authority to restrict the use of U.S. airspace and prevent the entry of aircraft into U.S. airspace.[54] Additionally, the FAA has the authority to prevent U.S. carriers and operators from flying to or within the airspace of other countries.[55] In regulating the use of airspace for the benefit of the public interest, the FAA must consider several factors as being in the public interest, including "assigning, maintaining, and enhancing safety and security as the highest priorities in air commerce" and "regulating air commerce in a way that best promotes safety and fulfills national defense requirements."[56]

During the current Ebola outbreak, the FAA has acknowledged its authority to restrict the use of U.S. airspace, but has cautioned that decisions made on a public health basis would involve other federal agencies.[57] The FAA has stated:

> While the FAA has the authority to direct flight operations in United States airspace, any decision to restrict flights between the United States and other countries due to public health and disease concerns would be an interagency decision that would engage the Departments of Health and Human Services/CDC, State, Homeland Security, and Transportation.[58]

CRS has been unable to identify any instances in which the FAA has restricted the use of U.S. airspace by incoming or outgoing flights purely on the basis of a public health concern.

### *Preventing Specific Passengers from Boarding Flights to the United States*

#### The "Do Not Board" List[59]

In recent years, federal agencies have developed a travel restriction tool to prevent the spread of communicable diseases of public health significance.[60] The public health Do Not Board (DNB) list was developed by the DHS and the CDC, and made operational in June 2007.[61] The DNB list enables domestic and international health officials to request that persons with communicable diseases who meet specific criteria and pose a serious threat to the public be restricted from boarding commercial aircraft departing from or arriving in the United States.[62] The list provides a tool for management of emerging public health threats when local public health efforts are not sufficient to keep certain contagious individuals from boarding commercial flights.[63]

In order to place a person on the DNB list, state and local health officials contact their local CDC quarantine station. The CDC determines if the person is (1) likely contagious with a communicable disease that presents a serious public health threat, (2) unaware of or likely not to comply with public health recommendations and medical treatment, and (3) likely to try boarding a commercial aircraft.[64] Once a person is placed on the DNB list,[65] airlines are instructed not to issue a boarding pass to the person for any commercial domestic flight or for a commercial international flight arriving in or departing from the United States. Other forms of transportation, such as buses and trains, are not covered by the DNB list. Once a patient is determined to be noncontagious, the CDC and the DHS must remove the person from the list, usually within 24 hours.[66]

#### Airline Corporate Policies[67]

Generally, airlines are under no legal obligation to provide transportation simply because a person has a valid ticket. As a matter of corporate policy, airlines have inserted clauses into their contracts of carriage reserving the right to deny transportation to any ticketed passenger under a number of circumstances, including passengers who may pose a safety risk to themselves, other passengers, or crew members. For example, United Airlines contract of carriage states the right to refuse transport to

> Passengers who are incapable of completing a flight safely, without requiring extraordinary medical assistance during the flight, as well as Passengers who appear to have symptoms of or have a communicable disease or condition that could pose a direct threat to the health or safety of others on the flight, or who refuse a screening for such disease or condition. (NOTE: UA requires a medical certificate for Passengers who wish to travel under such circumstances.... )[68]

Despite the existence of these contracts of carriage, in refusing to transport customers, air carriers must still abide by federal nondiscrimination laws, such as the Air Carrier Access Act (ACAA),[69] or risk civil penalties.[70] For more on these laws, see "Federal Nondiscrimination Laws."

The CDC has issued guidance to assist airline crew in identifying passengers who may be infected with Ebola before they board an aircraft.[71] This guidance provides that any passengers with certain symptoms and a history of recent travel in Guinea, Liberia, or Sierra Leone should be reported immediately to the CDC.[72]

### *Reporting Sick Persons Aboard U.S.-Bound Flights*[73]

Federal law requires an aircraft commander to immediately report to a CDC quarantine station nearest the port or airport of arrival if there is (1) a death on board or (2) any ill person among the passengers and crew.[74] These required reports are to be made to air traffic control and "[o]nce the FAA receives [the] report, it promptly communicates it to the CDC Emergency Operations Center."[75] Therefore, if the flight crew of a commercial aircraft arriving in the United States becomes aware of an ill person on board, which could include a person with EVD symptoms, federal law requires the flight's commander to notify the nearest quarantine station.[76]

The CDC has also issued guidance to instruct airline crews on managing ill passengers on board if Ebola infection is suspected.[77] It also provides guidance on cleaning aircraft to reduce the risk of spreading the disease, including recommending the use of personal protective equipment by cleaning crews.[78]

## International Health Regulations (IHR)[79]

### *Overview of the IHR*

In May 2005, the World Health Assembly adopted a revision of its 1969 International Health Regulations, giving a new mandate to the World Health Organization (WHO) and member states to increase their respective roles and responsibilities for the protection of international public health.[80] The IHR(1969) had focused on just three diseases (cholera, plague, and yellow fever). The IHR(2005) have broadened the scope of the 1969 regulations by addressing existing, new, and re-emergent diseases, as well as emergencies caused by non-infectious disease agents.[81] The IHR(2005) also include provisions regarding designated national points of contact, definitions of core public health capacities, disease control measures (such as quarantine and border controls), and others. The IHR(2005) require the WHO to recommend, and State Parties to use, control measures that are no more restrictive than necessary to achieve the desired level of health protection.

The IHR were agreed upon by a consensus process among the member states, and represent a balance between sovereign rights and a commitment to work together to prevent the international spread of disease. The IHR(2005) are binding on all WHO member states as of June 15, 2007, except for those that have rejected the regulations or submitted reservations.[82] While the IHR(2005) contain mechanisms, such as negotiation and arbitration, to assist States Parties in reaching mutually acceptable solutions where disputes arise, ultimately the IHR(2005) do not provide an enforcement mechanism to compel compliance with WHO provisions.[83] The United States accepted the IHR(2005) with three reservations, including the reservation that it will implement the IHR(2005) in line with U.S. principles of federalism.[84] Within five years of the entry into force date, State Parties must complete development of public health infrastructure that ensures full compliance with the regulations.

### *Public Health Emergency of International Concern*

Article 6 of the IHR(2005) requires member states to assess public health events within their jurisdiction and notify the WHO of any events that may constitute a Public Health Emergency of International Concern (PHEIC). Article 1 of the IHR(2005) defines a "Public Health Emergency of International Concern" as "an extraordinary event which is determined ... (i) to constitute a public health risk to other States through the international spread of disease and (ii) to potentially require a coordinated international response."

Cases involving certain diseases, such as smallpox and severe acute respiratory syndrome (SARS), automatically trigger mandatory WHO notification.[85] Whether reporting is required in the case of other diseases, including EVD, depends upon the seriousness of the public health impact, the unusualness or unexpectedness of the event, the risk of international spread, and the risk of international travel or trade restrictions.[86] On August 8, 2014, WHO Director-General Dr. Margaret Chan, upon the advice of the Emergency Committee, declared that the Ebola outbreak constituted a PHEIC.[87]

### *WHO Recommendations*

Under the IHR(2005), if the WHO director-general declares a "Public Health Emergency of International Concern," then the director-general must issue temporary recommendations, defined as "non-binding advice," which will depend upon the nature of the threat.[88] The IHR(2005) do not preclude State Parties from implementing measures that achieve a greater level of health protection than WHO temporary recommendations, provided that such measures are (1) otherwise consistent with the IHR(2005), and (2) not more restrictive of international trade and travel, and not more invasive or intrusive to persons, than reasonably available alternatives that would achieve the appropriate level of health protection.[89]

In the context of international travel during the current Ebola outbreak, the director-general recommended that in countries *with Ebola transmission*:

> There should be no international travel of Ebola contacts or cases, unless the travel is part of an appropriate medical evacuation.
>
> Confirmed cases should immediately be isolated and treated in an Ebola Treatment Centre with no national or international travel until 2 Ebola-specific diagnostic tests conducted at least 48 hours apart are negative;
>
> Contacts (which do not include properly protected health workers and laboratory staff who have had no unprotected exposure) should be monitored daily, with restricted national travel and no international travel until 21 days after exposure;
>
> Probable and suspect cases should immediately be isolated and their travel should be restricted in accordance with their classification as either a confirmed case or contact.[90]

For all other countries, the director-general recommended that "[t]here should be no general ban on international travel or trade."[91] Subsequent recommendations from the director-general provided that in countries with intense Ebola transmission:

> Exit screening in Guinea, Liberia and Sierra Leone remains critical for reducing the exportation of Ebola cases. States should maintain and reinforce high-quality exit screening of all persons at international airports, seaport, and major land crossings, for unexplained febrile illness consistent with potential Ebola infection. The exit screening should consist of, at a minimum, a questionnaire, a temperature measurement and, if fever is discovered, an assessment of the risk that the fever is caused by Ebola virus disease (EVD).[92]

# CIVIL RIGHTS

Governmental responses to infectious diseases, such as the current Ebola outbreak, may raise a classic civil rights issue: to what extent can an individual's liberty be curtailed to advance the common good?[93] As discussed above in the context of quarantine and isolation,[94] the United States Constitution provides for individual due process and equal protection rights, though these rights are not absolute and may shrink as the needs of the community grow. Aside from these constitutional issues, to what extent do federal nondiscrimination statutes protect individuals that may have been exposed to or diagnosed with Ebola in places of public accommodation and the workplace? Separate from the rights of sick individuals, may employers assert their right to dismiss individuals who are unable to report for work due to illness under an "employment at will" contract? Do certain employers, such as hospitals, have unique obligations under the Occupational Safety and Health Act to ensure that employees treating Ebola patients have a safe workplace? These questions are discussed in the sections below.

## Federal Nondiscrimination Laws[95]

Discrimination against individuals with an infectious disease may be covered by Section 504 of the Rehabilitation Act,[96] the Americans with Disabilities Act (ADA),[97] or the Air Carrier Access Act (ACAA).[98] The following sections discuss the status of individuals in three classes: individuals who may have been exposed to Ebola virus but are not sick; individuals who are sick with EVD; and individuals who have recovered from the disease.

### *Section 504 of the Rehabilitation Act and the Americans with Disabilities Act*

Section 504 of the Rehabilitation Act prohibits entities receiving federal funds from discriminating on the basis of disability. The ADA prohibits discrimination against individuals with disabilities in employment, state and local programs, public accommodations, and other areas.[99] Both acts use the same definition of an *individual with a disability*.[100] An *individual with a disability* is "[any] person who (i) has a physical or mental impairment which substantially limits one or more of such person's major life's activities, (ii) has a record of such an impairment, or (iii) is regarded as having such an impairment."

### *Qualifying As an "Individual with a Disability"*

It appears that the Rehabilitation Act and the ADA would most likely afford protection to two classes of individuals: ones sick from Ebola virus and those who have recovered from EVD. It is unclear whether the acts would protect individuals who may have been exposed to the virus but are not sick.

A symptomatic individual suffering from EVD would most likely qualify as an individual with a disability because EVD is limiting the major life activity of normal bodily functions. An individual who has recovered from Ebola would appear to qualify as an individual with a disability because he or she would be an individual with a history of EVD. It is not clear whether an individual who may have been exposed to Ebola virus, but is asymptomatic, would be covered by Section 504 or the ADA. It could be argued that such an individual qualifies because he or she is perceived as having Ebola. On the other hand it could be argued that he or she does not qualify because he or she is not perceived as having Ebola but is perceived to be a vector for the virus. Because there are no reported court decisions on whether an individual who is contagious but has no impairment qualifies as an individual with a disability, it is not possible to know whether an individual who is regarded as being contagious, but is not, would qualify as an "individual with a disability" or as an individual "regarded as" having a disability.

### *The Rehabilitation Act and Contagious Diseases*

Neither the Rehabilitation Act nor the ADA specifically discusses contagious diseases. The Supreme Court dealt with the issue in the context of

Section 504 in *School Board of Nassau County v. Arline*.[101] The Court considered the case of an elementary school teacher with recurrent tuberculosis who was terminated from her employment. She claimed she was dismissed because of a disability in violation of Section 504. The school district claimed she was terminated not because of her disability, but because she was contagious and posed a risk to others.

The Court first held that a contagious disease can qualify as a disability under the Rehabilitation Act, but noted that in most cases, a court must undertake an individualized inquiry into whether the plaintiff was otherwise qualified for her job to protect individuals with disabilities from "deprivation based on prejudice, stereotypes, or unfounded fear, while giving appropriate weight to such legitimate concerns ... as avoiding exposing others to significant health and safety risks."[102] The Court adopted the test proposed by the American Medical Association to determine whether an employee presents a significant risk to others. The Court held that the factors which must be considered include

> findings of facts, based on reasonable medical judgments given the state of medical knowledge about (a) the nature of the risk (how the disease is transmitted), (b) the duration of the risk (how long is the carrier infectious), (c) the severity of the risk (what is the potential harm to third parties) and (d) the probabilities the disease will be transmitted and will cause varying degrees of harm.[103]

The Court emphasized that courts "normally should defer to the reasonable medical judgments of public health officials."[104]

### *The ADA and Contagious Diseases*

The ADA does not specifically address individuals with contagious diseases, but it addresses individuals with disabilities who pose a "direct threat" to others. Under Title I, an employer may take otherwise prohibited actions against an individual with a disability if the individual poses a "direct threat." The term *direct threat* means "a significant risk to the health or safety of others that cannot be eliminated by reasonable accommodation."[105] Equal Employment Opportunity Commission regulations determine "direct threat" considering the following factors, based on reasonable medical judgment that relies on the most current medical knowledge and/or the best available objective evidence: the duration of the risk; the nature and severity of the potential harm; the likelihood that the potential harm will occur; and the imminence of the potential harm.[106] Under Title III, which prohibits discrimination in public accommodations and services operated by private entities, a business may deny accommodations or services to an individual with a disability who presents a "direct threat to the health or safety of others."[107] *Direct threat* is defined here to mean "a significant risk to the health or safety of others that cannot be eliminated by a modification of policies, practices, or procedures or by the provision of auxiliary aids or services."[108] Although Title II, governing state and local programs, contains no "direct threat" language, the Department of Justice has interpreted language in Title II to provide the same "direct threat" allowances and requirements as Title III.[109]

An individual sick with EVD who is symptomatic and contagious would probably be found to represent a direct threat to others in close proximity. Therefore, under the ADA, an employer, a business, or a state or local program could take steps to protect others from the contagious individual. However, individuals who are not contagious would probably not represent a direct threat to others. Accordingly, it appears that employers could not act adversely against such individuals, and businesses and state and local programs would need to give such individuals full access under the ADA.

### *The Air Carrier Access Act*[110]

The Air Carrier Access Act (ACAA) prohibits discrimination by air carriers against "otherwise qualified individual[s]" on the basis of disability.[111] Enacted in 1986, prior to the ADA, the law currently applies to foreign carriers, with respect to flights that begin or end at a U.S. airport, and U.S. carriers, with some exceptions.[112] Generally, the law prohibits the exclusion of qualified individuals with a disability from air transportation or related services, except when specifically permitted under the regulations.[113] The regulations specifically address when it is permissible to exclude a passenger with a communicable disease.[114] Under the regulations, carriers are prohibited from taking the following actions on the basis that a passenger has a communicable disease, *unless* the passenger's condition poses a direct threat:

- refusing to provide transportation;
- delaying the passenger's transportation, for example, by requiring the passenger to take a later flight;
- imposing any condition, restriction, or requirement not imposed on other passengers; or
- requiring the passenger to provide a medical certificate.[115]

The passenger's condition is a direct threat if it poses a "significant risk to the health or safety of others that cannot be eliminated by a modification of policies, practices, or procedures, or by the provision of auxiliary aids or services."[116] In determining whether a direct threat exists, the carrier is required to make an individualized assessment, "based on reasonable judgment that relies on current medical knowledge or on the best available objective evidence."[117] In making this individualized assessment, the carrier may rely on "directives issued by public health authorities," including the CDC.[118] If a carrier determines that a passenger poses a direct threat, the carrier must select the "least restrictive response from the point of view of the passenger, consistent with protecting the health and safety of others."[119] Carriers that violate the ACAA may be subject to civil penalty, levied by the Department of Transportation after notice and an opportunity for a hearing.[120]

## Employment Issues[121]

As discussed above,[122] the use of various infection control measures, such as quarantine and isolation, is a critical component of government efforts to minimize the possible spread of Ebola. In 2006, in response to the threat of pandemic influenza, the Homeland Security Council prepared an implementation plan that described more than 300 critical actions, including quarantine and isolation, that could be used to respond to a potential outbreak of contagious disease.[123]

While quarantine and isolation could prove to be effective for minimizing Ebola exposure, they may also raise various employment concerns, particularly for those workers who fear losing their jobs or wages if they are forced to comply with a quarantine or isolation order. Tort law may provide some relief for workers who are terminated while they are quarantined or isolated. Infected workers may also be protected under the Family and Medical Leave Act if it can be established that they have a serious health condition. Finally, some jurisdictions have established employment protections for workers if a quarantine or isolation is ordered. The following sections review these topics in greater detail.

### *Wrongful Discharge in Violation of Public Policy*

The employment-at-will doctrine governs the employment relationship between an employer and employee for most workers in the private sector. An employee who does not work pursuant to an employment contract, including a collective bargaining agreement that may permit termination only for cause or identify a procedure for dismissals, may be terminated for any reason at any time.

Although the employment-at-will doctrine provides the default rule for most employees, it has been eroded to some degree by the recognition of certain wrongful discharge claims brought against employers. In general, these wrongful discharge claims assert tort theories against the employer. A cause of action for wrongful discharge in violation of public policy is one such claim. If isolation or quarantine were used to attempt to limit the spread of Ebola and an employee were terminated because of absence from the workplace, a claim for wrongful discharge in violation of public policy might arise.

A claim for wrongful discharge in violation of public policy is grounded in the belief that the law should not allow an employee to be dismissed for engaging in an activity that is beneficial to the public welfare. In general, the claims encompass four categories of conduct:

- refusing to commit unlawful acts (e.g., refusing to commit perjury when the government is investigating the employer for wrongdoing);
- exercising a statutory right (e.g., filing a claim for workers' compensation, reporting unfair labor practices);
- fulfilling a public obligation (e.g., serving on jury duty); and
- whistleblowing.[124]

Although most states appear to recognize a claim for wrongful discharge in violation of public policy, it is possible that a state may allow a claim only under certain circumstances. For example, Texas recognizes such a claim only if an employee is terminated for refusing to perform an illegal act or inquiring into the legality of an instruction from the employer.[125]

While the four categories of conduct identified above represent the classic fact patterns for a claim of wrongful discharge in violation of public policy, other actions could be deemed beneficial to the public welfare and result in a wrongful discharge claim if an employee is terminated for engaging in such actions. Some courts have broadly defined what constitutes "public policy." For example, in *Palmateer v. International Harvester Co.*, the Illinois Supreme Court indicated that

> [t]here is no precise definition of the term. In general, it can be said that public policy concerns what is right and just and what affects the citizens of the State collectively. It is to be found in the State's

constitution and statutes and, when they are silent, in its judicial decisions.[126]

Similarly, in *Boyle v. Vista Eyewear, Inc.*, the Missouri Court of Appeals stated that public policy "is that principle of law which holds that no one can lawfully do that which tends to be injurious to the public or against the public good."[127] These broad definitions suggest that an employee's isolation or quarantine during a pandemic in some states could possibly provide a public policy exception to the at-will rule of employment. It would seem possible for a court to conclude that the isolation or quarantine of individuals during a pandemic serves the public good and that the termination of individuals who are isolated or quarantined violates public policy. Some observers insist, however, that no court has ever held that it violates public policy to discharge an individual because he or she missed work because of a quarantine.[128]

If the government were to mandate individuals to isolate or quarantine themselves either because they were infected or because of the risk of infection, it would seem possible that such an action might constitute a strong argument for the public policy exception to the at-will rule of employment. In such case, the government would appear to be identifying a significant policy that would benefit the public good. Even if the government merely recommended isolation or quarantine rather than mandated such actions, an argument for a public policy exception to the at-will rule would still seem possible.

### *The Family and Medical Leave Act*

The Family and Medical Leave Act (FMLA)[129] guarantees an eligible employee 12 workweeks of unpaid leave during any 12-month period for one or more of the following reasons:

- the birth of a son or daughter of the employee and to care for such son or daughter;
- the placement of a son or daughter with the employee for adoption or foster care;
- to care for a spouse or a son, daughter, or parent of the employee, if such spouse, son, daughter, or parent has a serious health condition;
- a serious health condition that makes the employee unable to perform the functions of the position of such employee; and
- any qualifying exigency arising out of the fact that the spouse or a son, daughter, or parent of the employee is on covered active duty in

the Armed Forces or has been notified of an impending call or order to covered active duty in the Armed Forces.[130]

The FMLA applies to any employer in the private sector that engages in commerce, or in any industry or activity affecting commerce, and that has at least 50 employees who are employed for each working day during each of 20 or more calendar workweeks in the current or preceding calendar year.[131] To be eligible for family and medical leave benefits, an individual must have been employed for at least 12 months by the employer from whom leave is requested, and must have been employed for at least 1,250 hours of service with such employer during the previous 12-month period.[132]

The FMLA also covers public agencies, including federal, state, and local governments.[133] Unlike employers in the private sector, public employers do not have to employ at least 50 employees to be subject to the FMLA. Employees of public agencies, however, must have worked, generally for a specified number of weeks, to be eligible for benefits.

It seems possible that the FMLA might provide infected employees and employees who care for certain infected relatives with the opportunity to be absent from the workplace. The FMLA defines a *serious health condition* to mean "an illness, injury, impairment, or physical or mental condition" that involves either "inpatient care in a hospital, hospice, or residential medical care facility; or ... continuing treatment by a health care provider."[134] An employee who been exposed to Ebola may be found to have a serious health condition. If the FMLA's eligibility requirements were met, such an employee would likely be granted leave under the statute.

In addition, because the FMLA grants leave to an employee to care for a spouse, child, or parent with a serious health condition, an employee could be granted leave to care for a relative affected by Ebola if the employee met the statute's eligibility requirements. While on leave, the employee with the serious health condition or the employee caring for a spouse, child, or parent with a serious health condition could comply with a quarantine or isolation order without the fear of termination for at least 12 workweeks.[135]

An employee who was not exposed or who was not responsible for the care of an exposed spouse, child, or parent would not be protected by the FMLA. If such an employee sought isolation or quarantine to avoid exposure and was absent from the workplace, the FMLA would not prohibit the employer from terminating the employee.

### *State and Federal Laws Providing Employment Protections*

At least seven states, recognizing the lack of statutory protection for employees in a situation where isolation or quarantine may be necessary, have enacted legislation that explicitly prohibits the termination of an employee who is subject to isolation or quarantine. In Delaware, Iowa, Kansas, Maryland, Minnesota, New Mexico, and South Carolina, an employer is prohibited from terminating an employee who is under an order of isolation or quarantine, or has been directed to enter isolation or quarantine.[136] Under Minnesota law, an employee who has been terminated or otherwise penalized for being in isolation or quarantine may bring a civil action for reinstatement or for the recovery of lost wages or benefits.[137]

Two additional states have enacted legislation that addresses the treatment of employees who are subject to quarantine or isolation. Under New Jersey law, an affected employee must be reinstated following the quarantine or isolation.[138] Under Maine law, an employer is required to grant leave to an employee who is subject to quarantine or isolation.[139] The leave granted by the employer may be paid or unpaid.[140]

Although federal law does not protect from termination employees who may be absent from the workplace because of isolation or quarantine, there are examples of employee protections that are arguably analogous. The FMLA, for example, does grant leave to an eligible employee who has a serious health condition or who provides care to a spouse, child, or parent with a serious health condition. Moreover, an expansion of the FMLA to allow paid leave because of a serious health condition or to care for a spouse, child, or parent with such a condition has been proposed.[141] The availability of paid leave would likely minimize concerns about lost wages if an Ebola pandemic were to occur.[142]

The Uniformed Services Employment and Reemployment Rights Act (USERRA) provides another example of employee protection.[143] USERRA requires the reemployment of an employee who has been absent from a position of employment because of service in the uniformed services. USERRA and the FMLA illustrate Congress's awareness of events that may necessitate an employee's absence from the workplace.

### *The Occupational Safety and Health Administration*[144]

Employers whose employees could face workplace exposure to Ebola virus may be obligated to comply with applicable Occupational Safety and Health Administration (OSHA) requirements. OSHA, through enforcement of the Occupational Safety and Health Act[145] (OSH Act), is generally responsible for protecting workplace safety.[146] To this end, the act authorizes OSHA to promulgate workplace safety standards.[147] Employers that fall within the scope of the OSH Act's—and, thus, OSHA's—jurisdiction[148] must comply with these standards.[149] It appears as though the three primary OSHA-created standards that could apply to employee exposure to Ebola in the workplace are (1) the Bloodborne Pathogens standard, (2) the Personal Protective Equipment standard, and (3) the Respiratory Protection standard.

When no OSHA standard applies to a workplace hazard, employers must comply with the OSH Act's catchall provision, known as the "General Duty Clause."[150] The General Duty Clause generally requires employers to provide workplaces that are free of recognized hazards.[151] Thus, employers must comply with OSHA standards for minimizing a workplace hazard that could expose employees to Ebola virus. However, when such a hazard has no applicable OSHA standard, the General Duty Clause seemingly requires employers to minimize the chance that the hazard will cause employees to contract Ebola virus. Noncompliance with OSHA-created standards and the General Duty Clause can generally lead to penalties against employers.[152] However, the OSH Act does not provide monetary relief to employees who are harmed by employer violations of OSHA standards or the General Duty Clause.

### *The Bloodborne Pathogens Standard*

The Bloodborne Pathogens standard appears aimed at preventing disease-causing microorganisms that are present in the blood—which, according to OSHA,[153] includes Ebola virus—from spreading to employees. The standard generally applies to employers with employees who could reasonably anticipate coming into contact with "blood or other infectious materials" during the performance of their workplace duties (e.g., hospitals).[154]

Among other things, employers that are subject to the Bloodborne Pathogens standard must have written plans for minimizing employee exposure to blood or other infectious materials, and such plans must be made accessible to employees.[155] Employers must review and update these plans at least once per year.[156] The Bloodborne Pathogens standard also contains "universal precautions," which seemingly require covered employers to manage employee behavior to help minimize the odds of employees coming into contact with infectious diseases.[157] For example, these universal precautions include having employees wash their hands with soap and water in certain circumstances;[158] properly dispose of used needles and other sharp medical equipment that has come into contact with human blood;[159] and refrain from eating, drinking, smoking, applying cosmetics, or handling contact lenses in areas where they can reasonably expect to come into contact with human blood.[160] The Bloodborne Pathogens standard further requires that employers provide "appropriate" protective equipment to employees that can be reasonably expected to come into contact with blood or other infectious materials.[161] Appropriate protective equipment is equipment that does not permit blood or other infectious materials to reach an employee's person or clothing.[162] Employers must provide such equipment at no cost to employees.[163]

### *The Personal Protective Equipment Standard*

OSHA's Personal Protective Equipment standard applies whenever personal protective equipment (PPE) is needed because of "hazards of ... environment ... capable of causing injury or impairment [to employees] in the function of any part of the body through absorption, inhalation, or physical contact."[164] This seemingly would encompass potential exposure to Ebola in the workplace as contact with bodily fluids that are infected with Ebola virus could cause employees to contract the virus. The protective equipment standard requires employers to assess their workplaces to determine whether hazards necessitating PPE are, or are likely to be, present.[165] Employers are then required to have affected employees use PPE that will protect against hazards identified during the assessment.[166] If PPE is required, the employer must generally provide such equipment at no cost to its employees.[167] However, there are exceptions wherein employees can be required to purchase their own protective equipment.[168]

### *The Respiratory Protection Standard*

OSHA has stated that when employees could be exposed to bioaerosols that contain Ebola virus (for example, when cleaning an infected surface with pressurized water could cause infected droplets to become airborne), employers must comply with OSHA's Respiratory Protection standard.[169] The Respiratory Protection standard requires, among other things, that employers provide affected employees with respirators when appropriate;[170] that covered employers develop and implement a written respiratory protection program containing worksite-specific procedures and requirements for employee respirator use;[171] and the selection,[172] fitting,[173] usage,[174] and maintenance[175] of appropriate respirators.

### *The General Duty Clause*

Under the General Duty Clause, employers must provide employees with "employment and a place of employment which are free from recognized hazards that are causing or are likely to cause death or serious physical harm." When no OSHA-created standard applies to a recognized workplace hazard but the hazard can cause employees to contract Ebola, the General Duty Clause may require employees to take precautions to reduce the likelihood that the hazard will cause employees to become infected with Ebola.

## End Notes

[1] For more detailed information on EVD, see CRS Report R43750, Ebola: Basics About the Disease, by Sarah A. Lister.

[2] Centers for Disease Control and Prevention, Cases of Ebola Diagnosed in the United States, available at http://www.cdc.gov/vhf/ebola/outbreaks/2014-west-africa/united-states-imported-case.html.

[3] Id.

[4] For a discussion of balancing individual legal rights and responsibility and communal objectives, see Institute of Medicine, Guidance for Establishing Crisis Standards of Care for Use in Disaster Situations (September 2009).

[5] This section was written by Jared P. Cole, Legislative Attorney. For a detailed discussion of quarantine and isolation, see CRS Report RL33201, Federal and State Quarantine and Isolation Authority, by Jared P. Cole.

[6] See Centers for Disease Control and Prevention, Quarantine and Isolation, http://www.cdc.gov/quarantine/.

[7] Id.

[8] U.S. CONST. art. I, § 8, cl. 3.

[9] 42 U.S.C. § 264(a).

[10] 42 U.S.C. § 264(b).

[11] See Exec. Order No. 13674, 79 Fed. Reg. 45671 (Aug. 6, 2014); Exec. Order No. 13375, 70 Fed. Reg. 17299 (April 1, 2005).

[12] Exec. Order No. 13295, 68 Fed. Reg. 17255 (April 4, 2003) (as amended by Exec. Order No. 13674, 79 Fed. Reg. 45671 (Aug. 6, 2014)). The diseases currently listed are cholera, diphtheria, infectious tuberculosis, plague, smallpox, yellow fever, viral hemorrhagic fevers (including Ebola), severe acute respiratory syndromes, and influenza viruses which have the potential to cause a pandemic.

[13] Control of Communicable Diseases; Apprehension and Detention of Persons With Specific Diseases; Transfer of Regulations, 65 Fed. Reg. 49906. Regulations regarding quarantine upon entry into the United States from foreign countries are also administered by the CDC, see 42 C.F.R. Part 71.

[14] See CDC Division of Global Migration and Quarantine home page at http://www.cdc.gov/ncpdcid/dgmq/index.html.

[15] CDC, "Quarantine Station Contact List, Map, and Fact Sheets," http://www.cdc.gov/ quarantine/quarantinestationcontactlistfull.html.

[16] 42 U.S.C. § 264(c).

[17] "Qualifying stage" means that such a disease is (1) in a communicable stage or (2) in a precommunicable state, if the disease would likely cause a public health emergency if transmitted to other individuals. 42 U.S.C. § 264(d)(2).

[18] 42 U.S.C. § 264(d)(1).

[19] Id.

[20] In response to the SARS epidemic, the Secretary of HHS in 2003 amended 42 C.F.R. §§ 70.6 and 71.3 to incorporate by reference Executive Order 13295, thus eliminating rulemaking delays for the publication of new diseases.

[21] 42 C.F.R. § 70.2.

[22] 42 C.F.R. § 70.3.

[23] 42 U.S.C. § 243.

[24] CDC, "Questions and Answers on the Executive Order Adding Potentially Pandemic Influenza Viruses to the List of Quarantinable Diseases," May 30, 2014, available at http:// www.cdc.gov/quarantine/qa-executive-order-pandemic-listquarantinable-diseases.html.

[25] Paula Mindes, Note, Tuberculosis Quarantine: A Review of Legal Issues in Ohio and Other States, 10 J.L. & HEALTH 403, 409 (1995).

[26] LA. REV. STAT. ANN. § 40:17(A). Exceptions are provided for certain diseases, including smallpox, cholera, yellow fever, bubonic plague, and tuberculosis. See La. Rev. Stat. Ann. § 40:17(B).

[27] Mindes, supra note 25, at 409. See, e.g., MD. CODE ANN., [Health] § 18-324, which formerly addressed only quarantine in tuberculosis cases. The governor may now exercise quarantine power during a "catastrophic health emergency" involving "deadly agents," which include "anthrax, ebola, plague, smallpox, tularemia, or other bacterial, fungal, rickettsial, or viral agent, biological toxin, or other biological agent capable of causing extensive loss of life or serious disability." MD. CODE ANN., [Public Safety] § 14-3A.

[28] Mindes, supra note 25, at 410.

[29] 219 F. Supp. 789 (E.D.N.Y. 1963).

[30] Greene v. Edwards, 164 W. Va. 326, 329 (1980).

[31] Jew Ho v. Williamson, 103 F. 10, 26 (C.C.N.D. Cal. 1900).

[32] This section was written by Michael John Garcia, Legislative Attorney.

[33] See, e.g., Landon v. Plasencia, 459 U.S. 21, 32 (1982) ("an alien seeking admission to the United States requests a privilege and has no constitutional rights regarding his application, for the power to admit or exclude aliens is a sovereign prerogative").

[34] Immigration and Nationality Act (INA) § 212(a)(1), 8 U.S.C. § 1182(a)(1).

[35] 42 C.F.R. § 34.2(b)(2) (defining a communicable disease of public health significance to include, inter alia, those diseases "listed in a Presidential Executive Order, as provided under Section 361(b) of the Public Health Service Act"). Ebola has been expressly listed by a relevant executive order since 1983. See Exec. Order No. 12452, Revised List of Quarantinable Communicable Diseases, December 22, 1983 (listing Ebola and other "Viral Hemorrhagic Fevers" as communicable diseases), revoked and replaced by Exec. Order No. 13295, Apr. 4, 2003 (continuing to specify Ebola as a communicable disease for purposes of Section 361(b) of the Public Health Service Act), amended by Exec. Order 13375, Apr. 1, 2005, and Exec. Order No. 13674, July 31, 2014.

[36] 42 C.F.R. § 34.2(b)(3)(i)-(ii) (including those diseases for which "a single case requires notification to the World Health Organization (WHO) as an event that may constitute a public health emergency of international concern, or ... [other diseases for which] the occurrence of which requires notification to the WHO as an event that may constitute a

public health emergency of international concern."). For discussion of WHO requirements concerning notification of Ebola infection, see infra at "Public Health Emergency of International Concern."

[37] Because of practical concerns, a foreign national arriving at a U.S. port of entry who is believed to have Ebola virus would be placed in isolation and given medical treatment, rather than immediately being placed in removal proceedings or given the option of promptly leaving the United States. For discussion of the isolation of arriving persons suspected of Ebola infection, see supra at "Federal Quarantine Authority."

[38] See INA § 101(a)(13)(C), 8 U.S.C. § 1101(a)(13)(C) (exempting most lawful permanent residents returning to the United States after briefly departing the country from being considered applicants for admission).

[39] See Jonathan Weisman, On Ebola Response, Congressional Republicans Put New Focus on Visa Suspensions, N.Y. TIMES, Oct. 20, 2014, available at http://www.nytimes.com/2014/10/21/us/on-ebola-response-congressionalrepublicans-put-new-focus-on-visa-suspensions.html?hp&action=click&pgtype=Homepage&version=HpSum& module=first-column-region&region=top-news&WT.nav=top-news&_r=1.

[40] See Jaime Fuller, The Ebola Travel Ban Is Really Politically Popular. Here's Why It's Not Happening, The Fix Blog, WASH. POST, Oct. 20, 2014, at http://www.washingtonpost.com/blogs/the-fix/wp/2014/10/20/the-ebola-travel-ban-isreally-popular-heres-why-its-not-happening/.

[41] INA § 212(f), 8 U.S.C. § 1182(f) (broadly permitting the President to "suspend the entry of all aliens or any class of aliens as immigrants or nonimmigrants, or impose on the entry of aliens any restrictions he may deem to be appropriate").

[42] A list of presidential proclamations pursuant to INA § 212(f) that are currently in effect can be viewed at http://travel.state.gov/content/visas/english/fees/presidential-proclamations.html. For further discussion regarding the potential use of INA § 212(f) to restrict the travel of foreign nationals from Ebola-stricken countries, see CRS Legal Sidebar WSLG1094, Can the President Bar Foreign Travelers from Ebola-Stricken Countries from Entering the United States?, by Michael John Garcia.

[43] Some federal courts have found that the right of an American citizen to return to the United States from abroad is a substantive due process right. See Fikre v. F.B.I., 3:13-CV-00899-BR, 2014 WL 2335343 (D. Or. May 29, 2014); Tarhuni v. Holder, 3:13-CV-00001-BR, 2014 WL 1269655 (D. Or. Mar. 26, 2014); see also Nguyen v. Immigration and Naturalization Serv., 533 U.S. 53, 67 (2001) (discussing privileges of U.S. citizenship, including "the absolute right to enter [the] borders" of the United States); Perez v. United States, 502 F. Supp. 2d 301, 306 (N.D.N.Y. 2006) ("a United States citizen cannot be barred from reentering the country").

[44] See infra at "Airlines and Travel Restrictions."

[45] This section was written by Alissa M. Dolan, Legislative Attorney.

[46] Press Release, "Statement by Secretary Johnson on Travel Restrictions and Protective Measures to Prevent the Spread of Ebola to the United States," available at http://www.dhs.gov/news/2014/10/21/statement-secretary-johnsontravel-restrictions-and-protective-measures-prevent [hereinafter DHS Ebola Press Release].

[47] Andrew Grossman, Carol E. Lee, and Jack Nicas, "U.S. to Check Temperatures of West Africa Passengers at Five Airports," WALL STREET JOURNAL, Oct. 8, 2014, available at http://online.wsj.com/articles/u-s-to-check-temperaturesof-west-africa-passengers-at-five-airports-1412788163.

[48] The only nonstop flights out of Guinea, Liberia, and Sierra Leone to Europe are operated by Air France (to Paris, France) and Brussels Airlines (to Brussels, Belgium). "Brussels Becomes Latest EU Airport to Screen for Ebola," Agence France Presse, Oct. 20, 2014. Both airlines are members of an airline alliance that includes a U.S. carrier; members of an alliance often coordinate their services and have codeshare agreements. Brussels Airlines is a member of the Star Alliance network, along with U.S. carrier United Airlines. Star Alliance, "Travel the World with the Star Alliance Network," http://www.staralliance.com/en/about/member_airlines/. Air France is a member of the SkyTeam network, along with U.S. carrier Delta Airlines. SkyTeam, "SkyTeam Members," https://www.skyteam.com/en/Aboutus/Our-members/.

[49] DHS Ebola Press Release, supra note 46; White House Blog, "Five U.S. Airports Are Enacting New Screening Measures to Protect Against Ebola," available at http://www.whitehouse.gov/blog/2014/10/08/five-us-airports-are enacting-new-screening-measures-protect-against-ebola.

[50] Press Release, "Enhanced Airport Entry Screening to Begin for Travelers to the United States From Mali," available at http://www.dhs.gov/news/2014/11/16/enhanced-airport-entry-screening-begin-travelers-united-states-mali. There are no direct flights from Mali to the United States. Id. Approximately 15 to 20 passengers whose travel originated in Mali arrive in the United States daily. Id.

[51] See, e.g., Convention for the Regulation of Aerial Navigation (Paris Convention), Oct. 13, 1919, Art. 1; Convention on International Civil Aviation (Chicago Convention), Dec. 7, 1944, Art. 1.

[52] 49 U.S.C. § 40103(a).

[53] 49 U.S.C. § 40103(b).

[54] See 49 U.S.C. §§ 40103(b), 44701. FAA issues Notice to Airmen (NOTAM) to announce temporary flight restrictions in U.S. airspace according to FAA regulation. See 14 C.F.R. §§ 91.137-138, 91.141, 91.143-145.

[55] See 49 U.S.C. §§ 40101(d)(1), 44701(a)(5). For an example of such a restriction, see "Prohibition Against Certain Flights Within the Territory and Airspace of Somalia," 72 Fed. Reg. 16710 (April 5, 2007).

[56] 49 U.S.C. § 40101(d)(1).

[57] Press Release, "FAA Statement on Ebola," Oct. 3, 2014, available at http://www.faa.gov/news/press_releases/ news_story.cfm?newsId=17375.

[58] Id.

[59] This section was written by Jared P. Cole, Legislative Attorney.

[60] For a summary of actions taken by DHS and the CDC to improve procedures to restrict persons with serious communicable diseases who intend to travel despite medical advice, see Public Health and Border Security: HHS and DHS Should Further Strengthen Their Ability to Respond to TB Incidents.GAO-09-58, October, 2008 [hereinafter GAO Public Health and Border Security Report].

[61] CDC, "Federal Air Travel Restrictions for Public Health Purposes—United States, June 2007-May 2008," Morbidity and Mortality Weekly Report, Sep. 19, 2008, available at http://www.cdc.gov/mmwr/preview/mmwrhtml/ mm5737a1.htm [hereinafter MMWR Report].

[62] Airlines also have general authority to refuse to board passengers with communicable diseases under certain circumstances pursuant to Air Carrier Access Act of 1986 (ACAA) and its implementing regulations. See 49 U.S.C. § 41705; 14 C.F.R. §§ 382.19, 382.21.

[63] The list, which applies to all citizens and foreign nationals, appears to have been developed under the general authority of the Aviation and Transportation Security Act of 2001, at 49 U.S.C. § 114(f) and (h).

[64] MMWR Report, supra note 61, at 1009.

[65] The Transportation Security Administration maintains the DNB list, which is separate from the No Fly List used to prevent known terrorists from boarding airplanes, but it serves a similar purpose. GAO Public Health and Border Security Report, supra note 60, at 29.

[66] MMWR Rep ort, supra note 61, at 1010.

[67] This section was written by Alissa M. Dolan, Legislative Attorney.

[68] United Airlines, "United Airlines, Inc. Contract of Carriage (Revised Nov. 7, 2014)" at 19, available at http://www.united.com/web/format/pdf/Contract_of_Carriage.pdf.

[69] P.L. 99-435 (1986), codified at 49 U.S.C. § 41705.

[70] See 49 U.S.C. § 46301(a)(1)(A).

[71] CDC, "Ebola Guidance for Airlines: Interim Guidance about Ebola Infection for Airline Crews, Cleaning Personnel, and Cargo Personnel," http://www.cdc.gov/quarantine/air/managing-sick-travelers/ebola-guidance-airlines.html [hereinafter CDC Guidance to Airlines].

[72] Id.

[73] This section was written by Alissa M. Dolan, Legislative Attorney.

[74] 42 C.F.R. § 71.21. For ships, the reporting requirement covers a death or illness that occurs within 15 days prior to the date of expected arrival or since departure from a U.S. port, whichever time period is shorter.

[75] Press Release, "FAA Statement on Ebola," Oct. 3, 2014, available at http://www.faa.gov/news/press_releases/ news_story.cfm?newsId=17375.

[76] CDC, "Quarantine Station Contact List, Map, and Fact Sheets," http://www.cdc.gov/quarantine/ quarantinestationcontactlistfull.html.

[77] CDC Guidance to Airlines, supra note 71.

[78] Id.

[79] This section was written by Edward C. Liu, Legislative Attorney.

[80] Fifty-Eighth World Health Assembly, agenda item 13.1, Revision of the International Health Regulations, May 23, 2005, at http://www.who.int/csr/ihr/en/.

[81] The full text of the IHR(2005) may be found at http://www.who.int/csr/ihr/IHR_2005_en.pdf.

[82] IHR(2005), Article 59.2.

[83] IHR, Article 56.

[84] HHS Secretary Michael Leavitt announced the acceptance of the IHR(2005) by the United States on December 13, 2006. See News Release at http://archive.hhs.gov/news /press/2006pres/20061213.html.

[85] IHR(2005), Annex 2.

[86] Id.

[87] WHO, "Statement on the 1st Meeting of the IHR Emergency Committee on the 2014 Ebola Outbreak in West Africa," August 8, 2014, available at http://www.who.int/mediacentre/news/statements/2014/ebola-20140808/en/. The continued existence of a PHEIC has been reaffirmed twice, on September 22, 2014, and on October 23, 2014. WHO, IHR Emergency Committee Regarding Ebola, http://www.who.int/ihr/ihr_ec_ebola/en/.

[88] IHR, Articles 1(1), 15(1).

[89] IHR, Article 43(1).

[90] WHO, "Statement on the 1st Meeting of the IHR Emergency Committee on the 2014 Ebola Outbreak in West Africa," August 8, 2014, available at http://www.who.int/mediacentre/news/statements/2014/ebola-20140808/en/.

[91] Id.

[92] WHO, "Statement on the 3rd Meeting of the IHR Emergency Committee on the 2014 Ebola Outbreak in West Africa," October 23, 2014, available at http://www.who.int/mediacentre/news/statements/2014/ebola-3rd-ihr-meeting/ en/.

[93] For a discussion of balancing individual legal rights and responsibility and communal objectives, see Institute of Medicine, Guidance for Establishing Crisis Standards of Care for Use in Disaster Situations (September 2009).

[94] See supra at "Legal Challenges to Quarantine."

[95] This section was written by Jane Smith, Legislative Attorney.

[96] 29 U.S.C. § 794.

[97] 42 U.S.C. §§ 12101 et seq.

[98] 42 U.S.C. § 1374(c).

[99] 42 U.S.C. §§ 12101 et seq.

[100] The Rehabilitation Act explicitly refers to the definition in the ADA. 29 U.S.C. § 705(B).

[101] 480 U.S. 273 (1987).

[102] Id. at 287.

[103] Id. at 288.

[104] Id.

[105] 42 U.S.C. § 12111(3).

[106] 29 C.F.R. § 1630.2(r).

[107] 42 U.S.C. § 12182(3).

[108] Id.

[109] 28 C.F.R. Part 35, Appx. A.

[110] This subsection was written by Alissa M. Dolan, Legislative Attorney.

[111] P.L. 99-435, 100 Stat. 1080 (1986), codified at 49 U.S.C. § 41705.

[112] 14 C.F.R. § 382.7.

[113] 14 C.F.R. § 382.11. "Individual with a disability" is defined as "any individual who has a physical or mental impairment that, on a permanent or temporary basis, substantially limits one or more major life activities, has a record of such an impairment, or is regarded as having such an impairment." 14 C.F.R. § 382.3. "Physical or mental impairment" is defined to include "any physiological disorder or condition... affecting one or more of the following body systems: neurological, musculoskeletal, special sense organs, respiratory including speech organs, cardiovascular, reproductive, digestive, genito-urinary, hemic and lymphatic, skin, and endocrine." Id. While no federal court has directly addressed the issue, this definition of "individual with a disability" appears to include individuals with communicable diseases. Under the ADA, courts generally accept communicable diseases as falling within the scope of "disability" if the diseases meet the same parameters that other physical and mental impairments must satisfy. See Bragdon v. Abbott, 524 U.S. 624, 631-42 (1998).

[114] 14 C.F.R. § 382.21.

[115] 14 C.F.R. § 382.21(a).

[116] 14 C.F.R. § 382.3.

[117] See 14 C.F.R. §§ 382.21, 382.19(c)(1).

[118] 14 C.F.R. § 382.11(b)(1).

[119] See 14 C.F.R. §§ 382.21, 382.19(c)(2).

[120] 49 U.S.C. § 463015.

[121] This section was written by Jon O. Shimabukuro, Legislative Attorney.

[122] See supra at "Quarantine and Isolation Authority."

[123] Homeland Security Council, National Strategy for Pandemic Influenza: Implementation Plan (GPO May 2006), available at http://www.flu.gov/planning-preparedness/federal/pandemic-influenza-implementation.pdf.

[124] See Steven L. Willborn et al., Employment Law: Cases and Materials 82 (1993); John F. Buckley and Ronald M. Green, 2010 State by State Guide to Human Resources Law 5-46 (2010).

[125] See Buckley and Green at 5-60.

[126] 421 N.E.2d 876, 878 (Ill. 1981).

[127] 700 S.W.2d 859, 871 (Mo. Ct. App. 1985).

[128] See Mark A. Rothstein and Meghan K. Talbott, Job Security and Income Replacement for Individuals in Quarantine: The Need for Legislation, 10 J. Health Care L. & Pol'y 239 (2007).

[129] 29 U.S.C. §§ 2601-2654. See also 5 U.S.C. §§ 6381-6387 (providing family and medical leave for civil service employees). For additional discussion of the FMLA, see CRS Report RS22090, The Family and Medical Leave Act: Background and U.S. Supreme Court Cases, by Jon O. Shimabukuro.

[130] 29 U.S.C. § 2612(a)(1). See also 29 U.S.C. § 2612(a)(3) (providing an eligible employee who is the spouse, son, daughter, parent, or next of kin of a covered servicemember with a total of 26 workweeks of leave during a 12-month period to care for the servicemember).

[131] 29 U.S.C. § 2611(4)(I). See also 29 U.S.C. § 2611(2)(B)(ii) (employers who employ 50 or more employees within a 75-mile radius of an employee's worksite are subject to the FMLA even if they may have fewer than 50 employees at a single worksite).

[132] 29 U.S.C. § 2611(2).

[133] See 29 U.S.C. § 2611(4)(A)(iii) (defining the term "employer" to include any public agency in accordance with Section 3(x) of the Fair Labor Standards Act, 29 U.S.C. § 203(x)).

[134] 29 U.S.C. § 2611(11).

[135] Although the FMLA allows for at least 12 workweeks of leave, it does not guarantee the payment of wages during such leave. Under Section 102(d)(2)(B) of the act, 29 U.S.C. § 2612(d)(2)(B), an employer may require the employee to substitute paid vacation or sick leave for the leave granted under the act. If such a substitution is not made, however, the employee is likely to be granted unpaid leave.

[136] Del. Code Ann. tit. 20, § 3136(6)(d); Iowa Code § 139A.13A; Kan. Stat. Ann. § 65-129d; Md. Code Ann., Health-Gen. § 18-906; Minn. Stat. § 144.4196; N.M. Stat. Ann. § 12-10A-16; S.C. Code Ann. § 44-4-530.

[137] Minn. Stat. § 144.4196.

[138] N.J. Rev. Stat. § 26:13-16.

[139] Me. Rev. Stat. Ann. tit. 26, § 875.

[140] The availability of wage or income replacement because of quarantine or isolation has been addressed by some commentators. See, e.g., Nan D. Hunter, "Public-Private" Health Law: Multiple Directions in Public Health, 10 J. Health Care L. & Pol'y 89 (2007). Many commentators maintain that existing wage or income replacement programs, such as unemployment and workers compensation, would probably not provide compensation for most employees affected by quarantine or isolation. Replacement wages were, however, reportedly paid during at least one quarantine. During the 1916 polio epidemic, quarantined families in the village of Glen Cove, NY, received replacement wages. See Guenter B.

Risse, Revolt Against Quarantine: Community Responses to the 1916 Polio Epidemic, Oyster Bay, New York, Transactions & Stud. of the College of Physicians of Philadelphia, Mar. 1992, at 34 ("Garbage cans were distributed free of charge, and quarantined families received replacement wages to compensate for loss of income").

With respect to the current Ebola outbreak, the governor of New York has also indicated that "any [quarantined] health care worker whose sponsoring organization does not [pay wages during quarantine], as well as adults who meet New York's criteria for quarantine, ... would be provided financial assistance for 21 days by the state." Governor Andrew M. Cuomo, New York State Releases Fact Sheet on State Screening Protocols at JFK International Airport, http://www.governor.ny.gov/news/new-york-state-releases-fact-sheet-state-screen ing- protocols -jfk-internationalairport. Disaster unemployment assistance pursuant to the Stafford Act may also be a possibility if it is determined that the act is applicable to an Ebola pandemic. See Federal Emergency Management Agency, Fact Sheet – Infectious Disease, available at https://www.fema.gov/media-library/assets/documents/ 99710; and CRS Report RL34724, Would an Influenza Pandemic Qualify as a Major Disaster Under the Stafford Act?, by Edward C. Liu.

[141] See, e.g., Family and Medical Leave Insurance Act of 2013, H.R. 3712, 113th Cong. (2013).

[142] Some states are exploring the availability of paid leave as part of their state disability insurance programs. In 2002, legislation that extends disability insurance benefits to individuals who are unable to perform their work because they are "caring for a seriously ill child, parent, spouse, or domestic partner" was enacted in California. See Cal. Unemp. Ins. Code §§ 3300-3306. Under the so-called Paid Family Leave Insurance Program, an individual who meets the program's requirements is eligible for benefits equal to one-seventh of the individual's weekly benefit amount on any day in which he or she is unable to perform the individual's regular or customary work. Similar legislation has also been enacted in New Jersey. See A. 873, 213th Leg., Reg. Sess. (N.J. 2008).

[143] 38 U.S.C. §§ 4301-4333.

[144] This section was written by Rodney M. Perry, Legislative Attorney.

[145] P.L. 91-596, 84 Stat. 1590 (1970). For general information on the OSH Act and OSHA, see CRS Report R43768, The OSH Act: A Legal Overview, by Rodney M. Perry.

[146] It is important to note that the OSH Act expressly allows states to control occupational safety and health regulation in certain circumstances. See 29 U.S.C. § 667. If OSHA approves a state occupational safety and health plan, which requires, among other things, that the plan provide health and safety protection that is at least as adequate as the protections provided by OSHA, see 29 U.S.C. § 667(c)(2), then the state plan requirements generally apply in place of OSHA's standards and regulations. 29 U.S.C. § 667(e).

[147] 29 U.S.C. § 655(b).

[148] The OSH Act expressly precludes its application to, and thus OSHA regulation of, certain employers. For example, the OSH Act does not apply to employment performed outside of U.S. states and territories, see 29 U.S.C. § 653(a); generally does not apply to federal, state, or local employment, see 29 U.S.C. § 652(5); and does not apply to self-employed individuals, see id.

[149] 29 U.S.C. § 654(a)(2).

[150] 29 U.S.C. § 654(a)(1).

[151] See 29 U.S.C. § 654(a)(1).

[152] See 29 U.S.C. § 666.

[153] "Ebola: Standards," https://www.osha.gov/SLTC/ebola/standards.html (last visited November 18, 2014).

[154] 29 C.F.R. § 1910.1030(b).
[155] 29 C.F.R. § 1910.1030(c)(1)(i); 29 C.F.R. § 1910.1030(c)(1)(iii).
[156] See 29 C.F.R. § 1910.1030(c)(1)(iv).
[157] See 29 C.F.R. § 1910.1030(d)(1).
[158] 29 C.F.R. § 1910.1030(d)(2)(iii)-(vi).
[159] See 29 C.F.R. § 1910.1030(d)(4)(iii)(A)(1).
[160] 29 C.F.R. § 1910.1030(d)(2)(ix).
[161] 29 C.F.R. § 1910.1030(d)(3)(i). Protective equipment includes, e.g., "gloves, gowns, laboratory coats, face shields or masks and eye protection, mouthpieces, resuscitation bags, pocket masks, or other ventilation devices." Id.
[162] Id.
[163] Id.
[164] 29 C.F.R. § 1910.132(a).
[165] 29 C.F.R. § 1910.132(d)(1).
[166] 29 C.F.R. § 1910.132(d)(1)(i).
[167] 29 C.F.R. § 1819,132(h)(1).
[168] See 29 C.F.R. § 1910.132(h)(2)-(h)(7).
[169] "Ebola: Standards," https://www.osha.gov/SLTC/ebola/standards.html (last visited November 11, 2014); OSHA, "Cleaning and Decontamination of Ebola on Surfaces," at 3 (2014), available at https://www.osha.gov/Publications/ OSHA_FS-3756.pdf.
[170] See 29 C.F.R. § 1910.134(a)(2).
[171] 29 C.F.R. § 1910.134(c).
[172] 29 C.F.R. § 1910.134(d).
[173] 29 C.F.R. § 1910.134(f).
[174] See 29 C.F.R. § 1910.134(g).
[175] 29 C.F.R. § 1910.134(h).

In: Ebola
Editor: MaryAnn Cole

ISBN: 978-1-63482-253-4


*Chapter 9*

# FEDERAL AND STATE QUARANTINE AND ISOLATION AUTHORITY*

***Jared P. Cole***

## SUMMARY

In the wake of increasing fears about the spread of highly contagious diseases, federal, state, and local governments have become increasingly aware of the need for a comprehensive public health response to such events. An effective response could include the quarantine of persons exposed to infectious biological agents that are naturally occurring or released during a terrorist attack, the isolation of infected persons, and the quarantine of certain cities or neighborhoods.

The public health authority of the states derives from the police powers granted by their constitutions and reserved to them by the Tenth Amendment to the U.S. Constitution. The authority of the federal government to prescribe quarantine and other health measures is based on the Commerce Clause, which gives Congress exclusive authority to regulate interstate and foreign commerce. Thus, state and local governments have the primary authority to control the spread of dangerous diseases within their jurisdictions, and the federal government has authority to quarantine and impose other health measures to prevent the spread of diseases from foreign countries and

---

* This is an edited, reformatted and augmented version of a Congressional Research Service publication RL33201, prepared for Members and Committees of Congress, dated October 9, 2014.

between states. In addition, the federal government may assist state efforts to prevent the spread of communicable diseases if requested by a state or if state efforts are inadequate to halt the spread of disease.

This report provides an overview of federal and state public health laws as they relate to the quarantine and isolation of individuals and a discussion of constitutional issues that may be raised should individual liberties be restricted in a quarantine or isolation situation.

## INTRODUCTION

In the event of a biological attack or the introduction of a highly contagious disease affecting the public, the U.S. health system may take measures to prevent those people infected with or exposed to a disease or a disease-causing biological agent from infecting others. The terms used to describe these measures, *quarantine* and *isolation*, generally apply to distinct groups of persons but are often used interchangeably. Quarantine typically refers to the "(s)eparation of individuals who have been exposed to an infection but are *not yet ill* from others who have not been exposed to the transmissible infection."[1] In contrast, isolation refers to the "(s)eparation of infected individuals from those who are not infected."[2]

Varying degrees of quarantine exist, and the authority to order quarantine or isolation is generally very broad. Primary quarantine authority typically resides with state health departments and health officials; however, the federal government has jurisdiction over interstate and foreign quarantine. In addition, the federal government may assist with or take over the management of an intrastate incident if requested by a state or if the federal government determines local efforts are inadequate.[3]

The variety of potential responses—from federal, state, and local authorities—implicates a number of legal issues. Namely, who is responsible for preventing an outbreak of the disease; and precisely what may be done? This report will examine federal and state authority to impose quarantine and isolation measures in order to prevent the spread of infectious disease.[4]

# FEDERAL AUTHORITY

## Quarantine and Isolation

Federal quarantine and isolation authority derives from the Commerce Clause of the U.S. Constitution, which states that Congress shall have the power "[t]o regulate Commerce with foreign Nations, and among the several states."[5] Section 361 of the Public Health Service Act (PHS Act) grants the Secretary of Health and Human Services (Secretary) the authority to make and enforce regulations necessary "to prevent the introduction, transmission, or spread of communicable diseases from foreign countries into the States or possessions, or from one State or possession into any other State or possession."[6] The law provides the Secretary with broad authority to apprehend, detain, or conditionally release a person. However, the Secretary may only exercise this authority in relation to communicable diseases published in an executive order issued by the President.[7] Executive Order 13295[8] lists the communicable diseases for which this quarantine authority may be exercised.[9] In 2000, the Secretary transferred certain authorities related to persons, including quarantine authority, to the Director of the CDC.[10] Both interstate and foreign quarantine measures are now carried out by CDC's Division of Global Migration and Quarantine.[11]

Generally, federal regulations authorizing the apprehension, detention, examination, or conditional release of individuals are applicable only to individuals coming into a state or possession from a foreign country or possession.[12] To facilitate containment efforts, federal regulations require airline pilots and ship captains to report immediately the presence of ill passengers on board their vessels.[13]

In addition, Section 361 of the PHS Act authorizes the apprehension and examination of

> any individual reasonably believed to be infected with a communicable disease in a qualifying stage[14] and
>
> (A) to be moving or about to move from a State to another State; or
>
> (B) to be a probable source of infection to individuals who, while infected with such disease in a qualifying stage, will be moving from a State to another State.[15]

If found to be infected, such individuals may be detained for such time and in such manner as may be reasonably necessary.[16] During times of war, the authority to apprehend and examine individuals extends to any individual "reasonably believed (1) to be infected with such disease [as specified in an Executive order of the President] and (2) to be a probable source of infection to members of the armed forces of the United States or to individuals engaged in the production or transportation of ... supplies for the armed forces."[17]

Regulations promulgated pursuant to this authority under the PHS Act may be found in Parts 70 and 71 of Title 42 of the Code of Federal Regulations. Part 70 applies to interstate travel, Part 71 to foreign arrivals.[18] The implementing regulations authorize the quarantine and isolation of individuals in order to prevent the spread of diseases identified in Executive Order 13295.[19]

In addition, pilots of both interstate flights and flights to the United States are required to report certain illnesses they encounter during flight in advance of their arrival into the United States to the CDC Quarantine Station closest to their destination airport.[20] There are currently 20 such stations operated by the CDC located at ports of entry into the United States.[21] While there are not CDC officials at every port of entry, various agencies in the Department of Homeland Security (DHS) are authorized to assist the CDC in "the enforcement of quarantine rules and regulations."[22]

The Director of the CDC is also authorized to take measures as may be necessary to prevent the spread of a communicable disease from one state or possession to any other state or possession if he determines that measures taken by local health authorities are inadequate to prevent the spread of the disease.[23] To prevent the spread of diseases between states, the regulations prohibit infected persons from traveling from one state to another without a permit from the health officer of the state, possession, or locality of destination, if such a permit is required under the law applicable to the place of destination.[24] Additional requirements apply to persons who are in the "communicable period of cholera, plague, smallpox, typhus or yellow fever, or who having been exposed to any such disease, is in the incubation period thereof."[25]

The Secretary is also authorized to bar the entry of persons from foreign countries where the "existence of any communicable disease" poses a "serious danger" of entering the United States such that "a suspension of the right to introduce such persons and property is required in the interest of public health."[26] A rule implementing this statutory authority was proposed in 2005, but was not adopted.[27]

The PHS Act and related statutes also authorize measures to aid or enforce a quarantine in the event of a public health emergency. Section 322(a) of the PHS Act[28] authorizes the PHS to care for and treat persons under quarantine. Such persons may also receive care and treatment at the expense of the PHS from public or private medical facilities when authorized by the officer in charge of the PHS station at which the application is made.[29] Section 311 of the PHS Act[30] provides for federal-state cooperative activities to enforce quarantines. The federal government may assist states and localities in enforcing their quarantines and other health regulations and, in turn, may accept state and local assistance in enforcing federal quarantines. Under the authority of 42 U.S.C. § 97, the Secretary may request the aid of CBP, the Coast Guard, and military officers in the execution of quarantines imposed by states on vessels coming into ports.

Criminal sanctions are prescribed for violations of federal regulations issued pursuant to Section 361 of the PHS Act.[31] Violation of a federal quarantine or isolation order is a criminal misdemeanor, and individuals may be subject to a fine of up to $100,000, one year in jail, or both; organizational violations may be subject to fines of up to $200,000 per event.[32] Federal district courts may enjoin individuals and organizations from violation of CDC quarantine regulations.[33]

## Do Not Board List

In recent years, federal agencies have developed a travel restriction tool to prevent the spread of communicable diseases of public health significance.[34] The public health Do Not Board (DNB) list was developed by DHS and the CDC, and made operational in June 2007.[35] The DNB list enables domestic and international health officials to request that persons with communicable diseases who meet specific criteria and pose a serious threat to the public be restricted from boarding commercial aircraft departing from or arriving in the United States.[36] The list provides a tool for management of emerging public health threats when local public health efforts are not sufficient to keep certain contagious individuals from boarding commercial flights.[37]

In order to place a person on the DNB list, state and local health officials contact their local CDC quarantine station. The CDC determines if the person is (1) likely contagious with a communicable disease that presents a serious public health threat, (2) unaware of or likely not to comply with public health recommendations and medical treatment, and (3) likely to try boarding a commercial aircraft.[38] Once a person is placed on the DNB list,[39] airlines are instructed not to issue a boarding pass to the person for any commercial domestic flight or for a commercial international flight arriving in or departing from the United States. Other forms of transportation, such as buses and trains, are not covered by the DNB list. Once a patient is determined to be noncontagious, the CDC and DHS must remove the person from the list, usually within 24 hours.[40]

In September 2008, the CDC released a report[41] in which it analyzed the first year's experience with the DNB list. According to the report, the CDC received 42 requests to add persons to the DNB list, all of whom had suspected or confirmed pulmonary tuberculosis.[42] The agency approved 33 of the requests, of which 28 were placed by public health departments in the United States, and 14 were placed on the list while they were outside of the country.[43] Two of the 33 persons placed on the DNB list attempted to evade the air travel restriction, and both were detained by border officials and taken to local hospitals for evaluation and treatment.[44] The CDC found that "[j]udicious use of the public health DNB list can obviate the human and economic costs associated with conducting contact investigations when people with communicable diseases travel on commercial aircraft."[45]

## State Police Powers and Quarantine Authority

While the federal government has authority to authorize quarantine and isolation under certain circumstances, the primary authority for quarantine and isolation exists at the state level as an exercise of the state's police power. CDC acknowledges this deference to state authority as follows:

> In general, CDC defers to the state and local health authorities in their primary use of their own separate quarantine powers. Based upon long experience and collaborative working relationships with our state and local partners, CDC continues to anticipate the need to use this federal authority to quarantine an exposed person only in rare situations, such as events at ports of entry or in similar time-sensitive settings.[46]

Although every state has the authority to pass and enforce quarantine laws as an exercise of its police powers, these laws vary widely by state. Generally, state and local quarantines are authorized through public health orders, though some states may require a court order before an individual is detained.[47] For example, in Louisiana, the state health officer is not authorized to "confine [a person] in any institution unless directed or authorized to do so by the judge of the parish in which the person is located."[48] Diseases subject to quarantine may be defined by statute, with some statutes addressing only a single disease, or the state health department may be granted the authority to decide which diseases are communicable and therefore subject to quarantine.[49] States also employ different methods for determining the duration of the quarantine or isolation period. Generally, "release is accomplished when a determination is made that the person is no longer a threat to the public health, or no longer infectious."[50]

One common characteristic of many state quarantine laws is their "overall antiquity," with many statutes being between 40 and 100 years old.[51] The more antiquated laws "often do not reflect contemporary scientific understandings of disease, [or] current treatments of choice."[52] In the past, state laws were often enacted with a focus on a particular disease, such as tuberculosis or typhoid fever, leading to inconsistent approaches in addressing other diseases.[53]

Until recently, despite the inconsistencies and perceived problems with such laws, state legislatures have not been forced to reevaluate their quarantine and isolation laws due to a decline in infectious diseases and advances in public health and medicine.[54] However, in light of recent threats and security concerns, many states have begun to reconsider their emergency response systems, including the state's authority to quarantine.[55] A review of quarantine authority was listed as a priority for state governments in the President's 2002 *National Strategy for Homeland Security*.[56]

Federal authority over interstate and foreign travel is clearly delineated under constitutional and statutory provisions. Less clear, however, is whether the state police powers may be used to restrict interstate travel to prevent the spread of disease.[57] In a public health emergency, federal, state, and local authorities may overlap. For example, both federal and state agencies may have quarantine authority over an aircraft arriving in a large city from a foreign country. Thus, coordination between the various levels of government would be essential during a widespread public health emergency.[58]

## LEGAL CHALLENGES TO QUARANTINE AUTHORITY

Public health measures in emergency situations, including quarantine, involve balancing the rights of individuals with the state's police power to protect the needs of the public health, safety, and general welfare. Historically, this balance can be seen in public health crises over the past century or so. The U.S. Constitution and federal civil rights laws provide for individual due process and equal protection rights as well as a right to privacy, but these rights are balanced against the needs of the community. However, classic public health measures such as quarantine, isolation, and contact tracing are, nevertheless, available in appropriate situations, and, as new or resurgent diseases have become less treatable, some of these classic public health measures have been increasingly used. Therefore, the issue of how to balance these various interests in a modern culture that is sensitive to issues of individual rights has become critical.[59]

Some courts have recognized an individual's right to challenge his or her quarantine or isolation by petitioning for a writ of habeas corpus.[60] Although the primary function of a writ of habeas corpus is to test the legality of the detention,[61] petitioners often seek a declaration that the statute under which they were quarantined is unconstitutional.

## Dormant Commerce Clause Challenges

In 1824, the Supreme Court in *Gibbons v. Ogden* alluded to a state's authority to quarantine under the police powers.[62] In 1902, the Court directly addressed a state's power to quarantine an entire geographic area in *Compagnie Francaise de Navigation a Vapeur v. Louisiana State Board of Health*,[63] where both the law and its implementation were upheld as valid exercises of the state's police power. A shipping company in this case challenged an interpretation of a state statute that conferred upon the state board of health the authority to exclude healthy persons, whether they came from without or within the state, from a geographic area infested with a disease.[64] The shipping company alleged that the statute as interpreted interfered with interstate commerce, and thus was an unconstitutional violation of the Commerce Clause. The Court rejected this argument, holding that although the statute may have had an effect on commerce, it was not unconstitutional.[65] In a subsequent case, the Court made clear that at least where Congress has not taken action, it is "well settled" that states may impose quarantines to prevent the spread of disease even though quarantines "affect interstate commerce."[66]

## Due Process Challenges

In general, courts appear to have declined to interfere with a state's exercise of police powers with regard to public health matters "except where the regulations adopted for the protection of the public health are arbitrary, oppressive and unreasonable."[67] For example, in *Miller v. Campbell City*,[68] an order to evacuate an area was issued due to leaking methane and hydrogen gases. After some residents from a subdivision in the area became ill, the county commissioners declared the subdivision uninhabitable. The plaintiff was arrested when he crossed the roadblock enforcing the quarantine in an attempt to return home. The Tenth Circuit Court of Appeals upheld a finding that the evacuation order was substantially related to the public health and safety, and found no evidence that the quarantine action was taken in bad faith or maliciously.[69] The court noted that the county needed to act quickly because of the potential danger, and did so "with appropriate concern for the situation and the interests of all involved."[70] The court therefore found that the plaintiffs were not denied substantive due process. The court also held that because the plaintiffs were given the opportunity to present their objections orally to the local authorities, and could have entered written materials as well, the protections of procedural due process were satisfied.[71]

Similarly, a federal district court in *United States v. Shinnick*[72] upheld the PHS's medical isolation of an arriving passenger because she had been in Stockholm, Sweden, a city declared by the World Health Organization to be a smallpox-infected area, and she could not show proof of vaccination.

Likewise, a state court in *People ex rel. Barmore v. Robertson*[73] refused to grant a habeas corpus petition for a woman who ran a boarding house where a person infected with typhoid fever had boarded. The woman was not herself infected with the disease, but she was a carrier and had been quarantined in her home. She argued that her quarantine was unwarranted because she was not "actually sick," though the court noted that "[i]t is not necessary that one be actually sick, as that term is usually applied, in order that the health authorities have the right to restrain his liberties by quarantine regulations."[74] In justifying quarantine under these circumstances, the court explained that because disease germs are carried by human beings, and as the purpose of an effective quarantine is to prevent the spread of the disease to those who are not infected, anyone who carries the germs must be quarantined.[75] The court found that in the case of a person infected with typhoid fever, anyone who had come into contact with that person must be quarantined to prevent the spread of the disease.[76]

More recently, a federal district court in New York dismissed a claim alleging violation of substantive and procedural due process by a plaintiff who was diagnosed with tuberculosis and confined to a hospital for a few days against his will.[77] The court cited to Justice Burger's concurrence in *O'Connor v. Donaldson*, which noted that, pursuant to its police powers, a "[s]tate may confine individuals solely to protect society from the dangers of significant antisocial acts or communicable disease."[78] However, at least one state court has ruled that when a state confines an individual in order to prevent the spread of disease, the state must provide the individual with procedural due process protections such as, *inter alia*, notice explaining the grounds for confinement, the right to counsel, and the right to engage in cross-examination.[79]

However, some courts have refused to uphold the quarantine of an individual in cases where the state is unable to meet its burden of proof concerning that individual's potential danger to others, or if a restriction is viewed as unreasonable or oppressive.[80] In *Wong Wai v. Williamson*,[81] the San Francisco Board of Health ordered all Chinese residents to be inoculated against bubonic plague and restricted their right to leave the city, citing nine deaths allegedly from plague. The inoculations were tainted, causing severe consequences. A court inferred that the regulations were properly authorized, but nevertheless struck them down as "not based on any established distinction in the conditions that are supposed to attend the plague, or the persons exposed to its contagions."[82] Shortly after, in *Jew Ho v. Williamson*, the same court noted that the quarantine requirements applied only to Chinese residents and questioned whether bubonic plague actually caused the reported deaths. It invalidated the quarantine because it was "unreasonable, unjust and oppressive" and constituted discrimination in violation of the Fourteenth Amendment.[83]

## Additional Potential Challenges

Additional legal issues might be raised if quarantine, isolation, and other public health measures were used to deal with a widespread domestic public health emergency. If government agencies requisition private facilities for quarantine purposes, such as in the case of overburdened medical facilities, the legal questions regarding eminent domain power may arise.[84]

A new development in the law relating to quarantine is the possible use of self-imposed or home quarantines. States may need to consider whether their ability to impose quarantine also includes the authorities necessary to support a population asked to voluntarily stay at home for a period of time.[85] Such authority may include the ability to offer legal immunity to businesses asked to provide facilities for quarantine.

# End Notes

[1] Homeland Security Council, National Strategy for Pandemic Influenza: Implementation Plan 209 (GPO May 2006) available at http://www.flu.gov/planning-preparedness/federal/ pandemic-influenza-implementation.pdf.

[2] Id. at n.207.

[3] 42 U.S.C. § 264; 42 C.F.R. § 70.2. During the 2003 outbreak of severe acute respiratory syndrome (SARS), U.S. patients were isolated until they were no longer infectious, allowing them to receive medical care and helping to contain the spread of the illness. However, there were no individual or population-based quarantines of persons who may have been in contact with infected persons. The CDC advised persons who were exposed, but not symptomatic, to monitor themselves for symptoms and further advised home isolation and medical evaluation if symptoms appeared. CDC, Isolation and Quarantine Fact Sheet, 2004, available at http://www.cdc.gov/ncidod/dq/sars_facts/ isolationquarantine.pdf.

[4] See generally CRS Report R40554, The 2009 Influenza Pandemic: An Overview, by Sarah A. Lister and C. Stephen Redhead; Homeland Security Council, National Strategy for Pandemic Influenza, (GPO November 2005), and Homeland Security Council, National Strategy for Pandemic Influenza: Implementation Plan (GPO May 2006).

[5] U.S. CONST. art. I, § 8, cl. 3.

[6] 42 U.S.C. § 264(a). Violation of federal quarantine and isolation regulations is a criminal misdemeanor, punishable by fine and/or imprisonment, 42 U.S.C. § 271. The statute also authorizes other public health measures, including destruction of animals or articles determined to be sources of communicable disease. 42 U.S.C. § 264(a). Originally, the statute conferred this authority on the Surgeon General; however, pursuant to Reorganization Plan No. 3 of 1966, all statutory powers and functions of the Surgeon General were transferred to the Secretary of Health, Education, and Welfare (now Secretary of HHS). In 2000, the Secretary of HHS transferred authority under this provision to the Director of the Centers for Disease Control and Prevention (CDC). CDC's Division of Global Migration and Quarantine carries out quarantine and related activities. http://www.cdc.gov/ncidod/dq/index.htm.

[7] 42 U.S.C. § 264(b).

[8] See Exec. Order No. 13674, 79 Fed. Reg. 45671 (Aug. 6, 2014); Exec. Order No. 13375, 70 Fed. Reg. 17299 (April 1, 2005).

[9] Exec. Order No. 13295, 68 Fed. Reg. 17255 (April 4, 2003). The diseases currently listed are cholera, diphtheria, infectious tuberculosis, plague, smallpox, yellow fever, viral hemorrhagic fevers (including ebola), severe acute respiratory syndrome (SARS), and influenza viruses which have the potential to cause a pandemic.

[10] Control of Communicable Diseases; Apprehension and Detention of Persons With Specific Diseases; Transfer of Regulations, 65 Fed. Reg.49906. Regulations regarding quarantine upon entry into the United States from foreign countries are also administered by the CDC, see 42 C.F.R. Part 71.

[11] See CDC Division of Global Migration and Quarantine home page at http://www.cdc.gov/ ncpdcid/dgmq/index.html.

[12] 42 U.S.C. § 264(c).

[13] 42 C.F.R. § 71.21. During the 2003 response to the severe acute respiratory syndrome (SARS) epidemic, federal officials provided health alert information to air travelers returning to the United States from areas with SARS outbreaks, boarded airplanes with travelers reported to be ill to assess their symptoms, and facilitated transport of ill passengers to hospitals.

Federal officials also provided updates to the public and worked with state and local public health agencies to investigate possible SARS cases. See Mark A. Rothstein et al., Quarantine and Isolation: Lessons Learned From SARS: A Report to the Centers for Disease Control and Prevention (2003) available at http://www.instituteforbioethics.com (hereinafter, Quarantine and Isolation).

[14] "Qualifying stage" means that such a disease is (1) in a communicable stage or (2) in a precommunicable state, if the disease would likely cause a public health emergency if transmitted to other individuals. 42 U.S.C. § 264(d)(2).

[15] 42 U.S.C. § 264(d)(1).

[16] Id.

[17] 42 U.S.C. § 266.

[18] In response to the SARS epidemic, the Secretary of HHS in 2003 amended 42 C.F.R. §§ 70.6 and 71.3 to incorporate by reference Executive Order 13295, thus eliminating rulemaking delays for the publication of new diseases.

[19] See 42 C.F.R. § 70.6 (interstate); 42 C.F.R. § 71.32 (foreign). The diseases currently listed are cholera, diphtheria, infectious tuberculosis, plague, smallpox, yellow fever, viral hemorrhagic fevers (including ebola), severe acute respiratory syndrome (SARS), and influenza viruses which have the potential to cause a pandemic.

[20] 42 C.F.R. §§ 70.4, 71.21(b). It appears as though pilots would report illnesses to the Federal Aviation Administration (FAA) Air Traffic Services Unit, which would then communicate with the CDC Emergency Operations Center. See Press Release, "FAA Statement on Ebola," Oct. 3, 2014, available at http://www.faa.gov/news/press_releases/ news_story.cfm?newsId=17375.

[21] See Centers for Disease Control and Prevention, U.S. Quarantine Stations available at http://www.cdc.gov/ quarantine/quarantine-stations-us.html.

[22] 42 U.S.C. § 268. HHS also works closely with the Department of Homeland Security (DHS) and its agencies. HHS and DHS signed a Memorandum of Understanding in 2005 that sets forth specific cooperation mechanisms to implement their respective statutory responsibilities for quarantine and other public health measures. Memorandum of Understanding Between the Department of Health and Human Services and the Department of Homeland Security, available at http://www.aclu.org/pdfs/privacy/hhs_dhs_mou.pdf. DHS has three agencies that may aid CDC in its enforcement of quarantine rules and regulations pursuant to 42 U.S.C. § 268(b). They are CBP, U.S. Immigration and Customs Enforcement (ICE), and the U.S. Coast Guard. In addition to DHS, CDC may also rely on other federal law enforcement agencies and state and local law enforcement agencies.

[23] 42 C.F.R. § 70.2.

[24] 42 C.F.R. § 70.3.

[25] 42 C.F.R. § 70.5.

[26] 42 U.S.C. § 265. Originally, the statute conferred this authority on the Surgeon General; however, pursuant to Reorganization Plan No. 3 of 1966, all statutory powers and functions of the Surgeon General were transferred to the Secretary of Health, Education, and Welfare. In 1979, the Department of Health, Education, and Welfare (HEW) was redesignated as the Department of Health and Human Services (HHS). P.L. 96-88, Title V., § 509. In 2003, the President's authorities under the original statute were delegated to the Secretary. Exec. Order No. 13295, 68 Fed. Reg. 17255.

[27] See Control of Communicable Diseases, Notice of Proposed Rulemaking, 70 Fed. Reg. 71892.

[28] 42 U.S.C. § 249(a).

29 42 U.S.C. § 249(c).

[30] 42 U.S.C. § 243.

[31] 42 U.S.C. § 271.

[32] See 18 U.S.C. §§ 3559, 3571.

[33] Federal district courts have jurisdiction over civil claims involving federal law. See 28 U.S.C. § 1331.

[34] For a summary of actions taken by DHS and the CDC to improve procedures to restrict persons with serious communicable diseases who intend to travel despite medical advice, see Public Health and Border Security: HHS and DHS Should Further Strengthen Their Ability to Respond to TB Incidents.GAO-09-58, October, 2008 [hereinafter GAO Public Health and Border Security Report]..

[35] CDC, "Federal Air Travel Restrictions for Public Health Purposes—United States, June 2007-May 2008", Morbidity and Mortality Weekly Report, Sep. 19, 2008, available at http://www.cdc.gov/mmwr/preview/mmwrhtml/ mm5737a1.htm [hereinafter MMWR Report].

[36] Airlines also have general authority to refuse to board passengers with communicable diseases under certain circumstances pursuant to Air Carrier Access Act of 1986 (ACAA) and its implementing regulations. See 49 U.S.C. § 41705; 14 C.F.R. §§ 382.19, 382.21.

[37] The list, which applies to all citizens and foreign nationals, appears to have been developed under the general authority of the Aviation and Transportation Security Act of 2001, at 49 U.S.C. § 114(f) and (h).

[38] MMWR Report, supra note 35, at 1009.

[39] The Transportation Security Administration maintains the DNB list, which is separate from the No Fly List used to prevent known terrorists from boarding airplanes, but it serves a similar purpose. GAO Public Health and Border Security Report, supra note 34, at 29.

[40] MMWR Report, supra note 35, at 1010.

[41] See generally id.

[42] Id. at 1010.

[43] Id.

[44] Id. at 1011.

[45] Id.

[46] CDC, "Questions and Answers on the Executive Order Adding Potentially Pandemic Influenza Viruses to the List of Quarantinable Diseases," May 30, 2014, available at http://www.cdc.gov/quarantine/qa-executive-order-pandemic-listquarantinable-diseases.html. The complexities of this shared power have been noted. One analysis observed that "When it comes to the exercise of isolation and quarantine powers, reality tends to be messier than the conceptual realm. Public health officials need clear lines of authority in emergency situations, often the moments when isolation and quarantine might be required. Unfortunately, confusion about which level of government should take the lead often occurs, thus revealing the ability of quarantine powers to spotlight difficulties federalism poses for public health." David P. Fidler, Lawrence O. Gostin, and Howard Markel, Through the Quarantine Looking Glass: Drug-Resistant Tuberculosis and Public Health Governance, Law and Ethics, 35 J. OF LAW, MEDICINE & ETHICS 616 (2007). Another commentator has noted that "Given the variation in due process rights in connection with quarantine, which may be afforded under federal and state law, one can foresee the possibility of considerable conflict." Felice Batlan, Law in the Time of Cholera: Disease, State Power, and Quarantines Past and Future, 80 TEMP. L. REV. 53, 119 (2007).

[47] Paula Mindes, Note, Tuberculosis Quarantine: A Review of Legal Issues in Ohio and Other States, 10 J.L. & HEALTH 403, 409 (1995).

[48] LA. REV. STAT. ANN. § 40:17(A). Exceptions are provided for certain diseases, including smallpox, cholera, yellow fever, bubonic plague, and tuberculosis. See La. Rev. Stat. Ann. § 40:17(B).

[49] Mindes, supra note 47, at 409. See e.g., MD. CODE ANN., [Health] § 18-324, which formerly addressed only quarantine in tuberculosis cases. The governor may now exercise quarantine power during a "catastrophic health emergency" involving "deadly agents," which include "anthrax, ebola, plague, smallpox, tularemia, or other bacterial, fungal, rickettsial, or viral agent, biological toxin, or other biological agent capable of causing extensive loss of life or serious disability." MD. CODE ANN., [Public Safety] § 14-3A.

[50] Mindes, supra note 47, at 410.

[51] Lawrence O. Gostin, et al., The Law and the Public's Health: A Study of Infectious Disease Law in the United States, 99 COLUM. L. REV. 59, 102 (1999). For a 50-state survey of quarantine provisions, see National Conference of State Legislatures, State Quarantine and Isolation Statutes, http://www.ncsl.org/research/health/state-quarantine-andisolation-statutes.aspx.

[52] Gostin, supra note 51, at 106106.

[53] Id. Following the SARS outbreak, some states had to quickly amend their public health laws to deal with that disease under their authorities.

[54] But see Edward A. Fallone, Preserving the Public Health: A Proposal to Quarantine Recalcitrant AIDS Carriers, 68 B.U.L. REV. 441, 448 (1988); Mindes, supra note 47, at 413 (citing Wendy E. Parmet, AIDS and Quarantine: The Revival of an Archaic Doctrine, 14 HOFSTRA L. REV. 53, 54-55 (1985)). No large-scale human quarantine has been implemented within the United States since the 1918 influenza pandemic, G. A. Gernhart, Forgotten Enemy: PHS's Fight Against the 1918 Influenza Pandemic. PUBLIC HEALTH REP. 559-561 (1999).

[55] Justin Gillis, "States Weighing Laws to Fight Bioterrorism," Washington Post, Nov. 19, 2001, at A01.

[56] Office of Homeland Security, National Strategy for Homeland Security, June 2002, http:// www.dhs.gov/sites/default/ files/publications/nat-strat-hls-2002.pdf.

[57] Rothstein, supra note 13, at 7-8 (discussing restrictions on travel to combat the spread of disease).

[58] Id. at 13 (suggesting that memoranda of understanding be developed between federal and state health officials setting forth responsibilities in cases of concurrent quarantine jurisdiction).

[59] For a detailed discussion of constitutional issues relating to quarantine see Michelle A. Daubert, Pandemic Fears and Contemporary Quarantine: Protecting Liberty Through a Continuum of Due Process Rights, 54 BUFFALO L. REV. 1299 (2007). For an analysis of how to balance the sometimes competing interests of personal and economic liberties with the public's health and security see Lawrence O. Gostin, When Terrorism Threatens Health: How Far are Limitations on Personal and Economic Liberties Justified? 55 FLA. LAW REV. 1105 (December 2003). See also David P. Fidler, Lawrence O. Gostin, and Howard Markel, "Through the Quarantine Looking Glass: Drug-Resistant Tuberculosis and Public Health Governance, Law and Ethics," 35 J. OF LAW, MEDICINE & ETHICS 616 (2007), where the authors note that courts have set four limits on isolation and quarantine authority: the subject must actually be infectious or have been exposed to infectious disease; the subject must be placed in a safe and habitable environment; the authority must be exercised in a non-discriminatory manner; and there must be procedural due process.

[60] Ex parte Hardcastle, 208 S.W. 531(Tex. Crim. App. 1919).

[61] Habeas corpus is "the name given to a variety of writs, having for their object to bring a party before a court or judge. In common usage, and whenever these words are used alone, they are usually understood to mean the habeas corpus ad subjiciendum." Specifically, habeas corpus ad subjiciendum is "a writ directed to the person detaining another, and commanding him to produce the body of the prisoner, or person detained. This is the most common form of habeas corpus writ, the purpose of which is to test the legality of the detention or imprisonment; not whether he is guilty or innocent." Black's Law Dictionary, 6th Edition, 1990.

[62] Gibbons v. Ogden, 22 U.S. 1, 18 (1824).

[63] 186 U.S. 380 (1902).

[64] Id. at 384.

[65] Id. at 387. See also Morgan's Steamship Company v. Louisiana Board of Health, 118 U.S. 455 (1886).

[66] Oregon-Washington R. & Nav. Co. v. State of Washington, 270 U.S. 87, 93 (1926); see O'Connor v. Donaldson, 422 U.S. 563, 582-83 (1975) (Burger, J., concurring) ("There can be little doubt that in the exercise of its police power a State may confine individuals solely to protect society from the dangers of significant antisocial acts or communicable disease").

[67] People ex. rel. Barmore v. Robertson, 134 N.E. 815, 817 (citations omitted) (Ill.1922); see also Zemel v. Rusk, 381 U.S. 1, 15 (1965) (the right to travel "does not mean that areas ravaged by flood, fire or pestilence cannot be quarantined when it can be demonstrated that unlimited travel to the area would directly and materially interfere with the safety and welfare of the area.").

[68] 945 F.2d 348 (10th Cir. 1991).

[69] Id. at 354.

[70] Id.

[71] Id.

[72] 219 F. Supp. 789 (E.D.N.Y. 1963).

[73] 134 N.E. 815 (Ill.1922).

[74] Id. at 819.

[75] Id. at 819-20.

[76] Id. at 820.

[77] Best v. Bellevue Hosp. Ctr., 03CIV.365(RMB)(JCF), 2003 WL 21767656 (S.D.N.Y. July 30, 2003) aff'd in part, vacated in part, remanded sub nom. Best v. Bellevue Hosp. New York, NY, 115 F. App'x 459 (2d Cir. 2004).

[78] O'Connor v. Donaldson, 422 U.S. 563, 582-83 (1975) (Burger, J., concurring).

[79] Greene v. Edwards, 164 W. Va. 326, 329 (1980).

[80] See State v. Snow, 324 S.W.2d 532 (Ark. 1959), where the court found insufficient evidence to show a person who had tuberculosis was in an active and communicable stage so that he could be involuntarily isolated. On the other hand, see City of New York v. Antoinette, R.., 630 N.Y.S. 2d 1008 (N.Y. Sup. Ct. 1995), wherein the court upheld detaining a tuberculosis patient in a hospital setting until the patient completed an appropriate course of medication.

[81] 103 F. Rep. 10 (1900).

[82] Id. at 15.

[83] Jew Ho v. Williamson, 103 F. 10, 26 (C.C.N.D. Cal. 1900).

[84] Compelled public use of private property in a public health emergency is not unheard of. "In Paris, in August 2003, after 11,000 deaths were caused by a heat wave, the government took over refrigerated warehouses and similar facilities to use them as temporary morgues." Rothstein, Quarantine and Isolation, supra note 13, at 42. Compensation may be appropriate

in some circumstances, but following a volcanic eruption, the State of Washington successfully argued that continued restricted access to a town near the volcano was a permissible exercise of police power and did not require compensation. Cougar Business Owners Assn. v. State of Washington, 647 P.2d 481, 486 (Sup. Ct. Wash. 1982). See David G. Tucker and Alfred O. Bragg, III, Florida's Law of Storms: Emergency Management, Local Government, and the Police Power, 30 STETSON L. REV. 837 (2001).

[85] Federal and state authorities generally provide for the care of persons mandatorily quarantined (see 42 U.S.C. § 249), but voluntary home-quarantine situations may pose new issues. See Steven D. Gravely, et al., Emergency Prepared ness and Response: Legal Issues in a Changing World, 17 THE HEALTH LAWYER 1 (June 2005).

# INDEX

## B



## C

## D



## E

## F

## G



## H

## M



## N



## O

## P



## Q



## R